Peer Support Services Reaching People with Schizophrenia

Megan Evans

Peer Support Services Reaching People with Schizophrenia

Considerations for Research and Practice

Springer

Megan Evans
Department of Psychiatry
Yale University
New Haven, CT, USA

ISBN 978-3-031-29041-1 ISBN 978-3-031-29042-8 (eBook)
https://doi.org/10.1007/978-3-031-29042-8

This Springer imprint is published by the registered company Springer Nature Switzerland AG
The registered company address is: Gewerbestrasse 11, 6330 Cham, Switzerland

For Andrew and Grace

Preface

Peer support, or non-clinical recovery support and services provided by people with lived experience of behavioral health conditions, is a rapidly growing field in behavioral health. With a rising need for behavioral health services and a shortage of workers, further expansion of the peer workforce is on the horizon. The nuances in the evidence base behind peer support, however, are complex. This book helps to clarify the varied intervention strategies and activities that make up peer support, its varied outcomes, and proposed intermediary links between intervention and outcome. While the material presented here is primarily focused on people diagnosed with schizophrenia or other serious mental illnesses, the lessons learned and implications for practice apply to a wider population of people with various behavioral health challenges.

This book is aimed at researchers and practitioners who are interested in deepening their knowledge of the complexities involved in peer support and peer-delivered services to inform research and service delivery. The book's focus on a particularly complex mental health issue, that of schizophrenia, is intended to illustrate that a holistic approach to care including peer support should be available to all mental health service users, including those diagnosed with the disorders that are most often considered severe. The book primarily uses the term schizophrenia in accordance with current diagnostic terminology; however, I acknowledge the heterogeneity in the term as well as criticisms of its reliability and validity.

Chapter 1 provides an overview of schizophrenia as a public health problem, and Chap. 2 outlines current approaches to treatment. Chapter 3 broadly summarizes some important theoretical bases of peer support and proposes a conceptual framework of the multiple inputs and outcomes of peer support at different levels of the socioecological model. A brief history of the modern recovery movement and the origins of peer support is detailed in Chap. 4. Chapter 5 reviews the evidence of peer support in mental health generally, and Chap. 6 presents the review methodology used to investigate its uses among people with schizophrenia specifically. Chapters 7 and 8 present the main findings: categorization of the varied components comprising peer support interventions and key issues in the field, respectively. Finally, Chap. 9 summarizes the findings and presents implications for research and practice.

New Haven, CT, USA Megan Evans

Acknowledgments

This book arose from my dissertation research completed at the Gillings School of Global Public Health at the University of North Carolina at Chapel Hill. I would like to thank the members of my dissertation committee, Drs. Gary Cuddeback, Carol Golin, Kathryn Muessig, and Kim Strom, for their support and valuable feedback. I would like to extend a special thanks to my mentor and dissertation chair, Dr. Edwin Fisher, for his unwavering support of this work and copious comments on earlier versions. I would also like to thank all the current and past members of the Peers for Progress research team, who collectively provided invaluable insight and feedback throughout this process. I would like to thank the team at the Program for Recovery and Community Health at the Yale School of Medicine for expanding my knowledge of recovery-oriented practice and critical perspectives on mental health. Finally, I would also like to thank the staff at Springer, in particular Megan McManus and Praveena John, for their help and support.

Contents

Abbreviations

ACT	Assertive Community Treatment
BMI	Body Mass Index
CATIE	Clinical Antipsychotic Trials of Intervention Effectiveness
CBD	Cannabidiol
CHW	Community Health Worker
CIL	Center for Independent Living
FEP	First Episode Psychosis
FGA	First-Generation Antipsychotic
HVN	Hearing Voices Network
IPS	Individual Placement and Support
MET	Metabolic-Equivalent Expenditure
mHealth	Mobile Health
NAMI	National Alliance for the Mentally Ill
NHS	National Health Service
PAD	Psychiatric Advance Directive
PORT	Patient Outcomes Research Team
RAMESES	Realist and Meta-narrative Evidence Synthesis: Evolving Standards
RCT	Randomized Controlled Trial
SAMHSA	Substance Abuse and Mental Health Services Administration
SGA	Second-Generation Antipsychotic
SMI	Serious Mental Illness
THC	Δ-9-Tetrahydrocannabinol

Chapter 1
Schizophrenia as a Public Health Problem

Schizophrenia is conceptualized as a mental disorder characterized by psychotic symptoms such as disorganization of thought and behavior, auditory or visual hallucinations, and paranoid and other delusional ideas [1]. In addition to these positive symptoms, the disorder is also characterized by negative symptoms such as flat affect, poverty of thought or speech, and lack of interest, pleasure, or motivation [1]. It is also associated with broad cognitive impairment that affects both social and nonsocial cognition [2]. Impaired social cognition manifests in difficulties identifying emotions, connecting with other people, inferring other people's thoughts, and reacting emotionally to others [3]. People experiencing schizophrenia often have difficulty interpreting social cues that allow people to gauge another person's moods and intentions [3]. These social deficits in cognitive functioning are associated with decreased community functioning [4].

The category of schizophrenia-spectrum disorders outlined in the fifth edition of the Diagnostic and Statistical Manual of Mental Disorders (DSM-V) includes the following diagnoses: schizophrenia, schizophreniform disorder, schizoaffective disorder, delusional disorder, brief psychotic disorder, and psychotic disorder-not otherwise specified [5]. This book primarily uses the term schizophrenia; however, I acknowledge the considerable heterogeneity in the term [6] and criticism of its limited reliability and validity [7]. As such, the information presented here is intended to translate to all mental disorders involving the experience of psychosis.

1.1 Complex Etiology of Schizophrenia

Although a variety of risk factors have been identified for schizophrenia and psychosis more generally, exact causes are far from understood [8]. Genetics have been implicated, with the strongest known predictor of risk identified as having a close biological relative who is affected [9]. Results from adoption and twin studies

M. Evans, *Peer Support Services Reaching People with Schizophrenia*,
https://doi.org/10.1007/978-3-031-29042-8_1

suggest that this familial clustering of psychosis is due largely to genetic factors [8]. It should be noted, however, that this interpretation of the evidence from twin and adoption studies is not without criticism [10]. Importantly, no single gene or genetic variant has been implicated as a necessary and sufficient causal factor for schizophrenia or psychosis [8]. Tremendous technological advances have enabled a proliferation of genomic research which has implicated over 100 independent genetic variants, both common variants and those that rarely occur [8]. Additionally, polygenic analyses across other conditions suggest that genetic loci contributing to schizophrenia risk are also implicated in other mental and physical illnesses [8]. A significant limitation of the current genetic research is that most studies have relied on ethnically homogenous samples of White people from European descent [8]. Thus, while genetics appear to play a role in the development of schizophrenia and other psychotic disorders, their role is complex, not fully understood, and certainly not a complete explanation.

A host of environmental factors are also significantly associated with schizophrenia and psychosis risk [8]. These risks exist across prenatal, perinatal, childhood, and adolescent developmental stages [8]. For example, inadequate nutrition [11], maternal anemia [12], exposure to heavy metals [13], and maternal stress [14] in the prenatal period are all associated with later development of schizophrenia. Obstetric complications [15], season of birth [16], and preterm birth [17] are perinatal risk factors for psychosis. Bullying [18] and maltreatment [19] in childhood are associated with development of psychosis, as are cannabis [20] and tobacco [21] use in adolescence. Minority status [22], income inequality [23], and low socioeconomic status [24] in any of these developmental stages are associated with a later development of psychosis [8]. Environmental risk appears to be cumulative [25] so that exposure to a greater number of environmental risk factors is associated with earlier age of onset [26, 27]. Additionally, there is likely significant gene-environment interplay implicated in the development of psychosis [8]. More research that thoroughly assesses both psychopathology and environment at multiple points during development will advance our knowledge of gene-environment causation [8].

Psychological risk factors for schizophrenia and psychosis are also important. Trauma plays an important role in the development of many mental disorders [28–30]; however, its role in the development of psychosis has historically been overlooked in favor of biomedical explanations [31, 32]. Nevertheless, the experience of childhood or developmental trauma has consistently been shown to be associated with later development of psychosis [33], and a dose-response relationship has been demonstrated, with those experiencing the most severe abuse being at the highest risk for developing psychosis [34]. Approximately 70% of individuals with early psychosis have a trauma history [35]. Developmental trauma has been shown to be associated with both positive [36, 37] and negative symptoms [37]. Furthermore, the experience of later re-traumatization is also associated with worsened symptoms of psychosis, and it is worth noting that most psychiatric patients suffer serious physical or sexual assaults in adulthood [38–40]. In addition, the very experiences of psychosis and psychiatric hospitalization can be traumatizing [41–43].

In sum, there are numerous and diverse factors that are associated with the development of schizophrenia and psychosis, and our understanding of causation is limited at best. However, the experience of psychosis is generally perceived to be caused mainly by biological and genetic factors, perhaps more so than any other mental illness phenomena [44]. While a biopsychosocial model of schizophrenia and psychosis is often emphasized, the reported ratio of biological to psychosocial etiology of psychosis studies is 16:1 [45], in effect reducing a complex, multilevel phenomenon to a simple, single-level issue [46, 47]. A more complete understanding of the etiology of psychosis necessitates further consideration of psychological and social factors.

1.2 Public Health Burden of Serious Mental Illness

Serious mental illnesses (SMI), including schizophrenia, pose a significant public health burden. The criteria for SMI diagnosis are having any diagnosable mental disorder, excluding developmental and substance use disorders, as well as experiencing serious functional impairment that is due to the illness and interferes with at least one major life activity [48]. Approximately 4–5% of US adults have an SMI [48], and proportions are similar in other countries [49]. SMI is commonly associated with diagnoses of schizophrenia-spectrum disorders, severe bipolar disorders, or severe major depressive disorders. However, any diagnosed mental illness that causes significant functional impairment and substantially limits major life activities can constitute an SMI.

The burden of mental illness is particularly concentrated among those diagnosed with SMI, making it a leading cause of disability [1]. In the United States, the associated per-person lifetime economic burden of SMI is estimated to be $1.85 million dollars, due to substantially worsened health outcomes, raised medical costs, and reduced economic outcomes across the lifespan [50]. People with SMI have a mortality rate 4.5 times greater [51] and an average life expectancy between 10 and 25 years shorter than that of the general population [52, 53]. People with SMI are more likely to die of unnatural and natural causes than people without mental illness [54]. Natural causes (e.g., cardiovascular disease) account for most of this excess mortality [51].

In addition to increased morbidity and mortality, people with SMI also disproportionately face economic and social problems. Compared to the general population, they have higher rates of unemployment [55–59], underemployment [56, 60], housing instability [61], and homelessness [62–64]. Strikingly, over a third of people with SMI earn less than $10,000 annually [55]. Over a lifetime, they earn half a million dollars less per person and spend 13 fewer years in full-time employment than those without SMI [50]. SMI is associated with a higher risk of incarceration [65, 66] and its estimated prevalence among jail and prison populations ranges from 15% to 30% [67–69]. Comorbid substance use disorders contribute to the overrepresentation of people with SMI in the carceral system [70]. Demonstrating the staggering incidence of incarceration among this population, people with SMI are jailed more frequently than they are hospitalized [71].

1.3 Public Health Burden of Schizophrenia

Schizophrenia considered alone also presents a significant disease burden and has enormous economic and social costs [72–74]. It is estimated that approximately 21 million people are living with schizophrenia, a number which is expected to continue rising with population aging and growth [72]. Despite affecting just 1% of the population, it is the 15th leading cause of disability worldwide [75]. Across several high-income countries, annual national costs associated with schizophrenia are estimated to be between US$94 billion and US$102 billion, with indirect costs contributing over half of the total costs [73]. Beyond economic costs, the humanistic burden is also of great concern. Schizophrenia is associated with decreased quality of life, comorbid depression, treatment side effects, and tremendous caregiver burden [74].

Furthermore, individuals experiencing schizophrenia have poor social and health outcomes. These include reduced social connections, reduced rates of employment, and an impaired ability to live independently [76]. Due in large part to the effects of deinstitutionalization, the criminalization of poverty and substance use, and an inadequate social safety net, people with schizophrenia disproportionately experience homelessness [77–79] and incarceration [69, 80]. Globally, people diagnosed with schizophrenia die between 13 and 15 years earlier than those without the disorder (Hjorthøj, Stürup, McGrath, & Nordentoft, 2017). Their risk of death is estimated to be between two and three times greater than that of the general population [81]. This reduced life expectancy can be attributed to unnatural (e.g., suicide) and natural (e.g., cardiovascular disease) causes [81]. Approximately 60% of all deaths among people with schizophrenia are due to natural causes [82]. Health behaviors such as smoking [81, 83], sedentary behavior [84], and substance use [82, 85] contribute to the heavy burden of mortality among people with schizophrenia. Furthermore, side effects of antipsychotic medications are known to be obesogenic and causally related to metabolic syndrome [81].

1.4 Substance Use Among People with Schizophrenia

Roughly half of people diagnosed with schizophrenia also have a comorbid substance use disorder, a rate that has not changed over time [86, 87]. The most common substances used by people with schizophrenia are the same as in the general population: nicotine, alcohol, and cannabis [74]. Nearly 60% of people diagnosed with schizophrenia currently smoke cigarettes, compared with just 15% among the general adult population [83]. Approximately a quarter have an alcohol use disorder at some point in their lifetime [86], and those experiencing severe psychotic disorders have four times greater odds of heavy alcohol use than the general population [88]. About a third of people with schizophrenia use cannabis [89] and a quarter meet the criteria for a cannabis use disorder [86]. Both rates are higher than that of the general population [90]. Here, the use of these substances is considered one by one; however, it should be noted that polysubstance use is common among this population [91, 92].

1.4.1 Nicotine and Tobacco Use

The use of tobacco among people with schizophrenia contributes greatly to the public health burden of the disease. For example, a large cohort study found that tobacco-related conditions were causally related to more than half of total deaths in people with schizophrenia [93]. Even so, this population is less likely to be screened for tobacco use in primary care [94]. Furthermore, smokers diagnosed with schizophrenia are less likely to receive cessation support from health professionals than smokers without schizophrenia [95]. The concern that smoking discontinuation might worsen the psychological condition of a person experiencing schizophrenia has not been supported by recent research [96–98]. Current guidance suggests that even patients with severe symptoms should be encouraged to reduce or quit smoking [99]. Approaches to smoking cessation for people with schizophrenia and other psychotic disorders should be designed with their unique needs and challenges in mind, as evidence shows that recent public health approaches to reducing smoking have not been effective among this population [88].

The relationship between smoking and schizophrenia is complex. It has been suggested that patients diagnosed with schizophrenia smoke in part to diminish negative symptoms of the illness, particularly anhedonia [100], as well as to mitigate the side effects of antipsychotic medications [74]. Biochemically, smoking could be viewed as an adaptive behavior as nicotine releases dopamine, while classic antipsychotics block dopaminergic transmission [101]. However, smoking is also associated with poor mental health outcomes. For example, among people experiencing a first episode of psychosis (FEP), cigarette smoking has been linked to higher ratings of psychiatric symptoms and functional impairment, lower medication adherence, and lower quality of life [102]. Aside from the mental health impacts, over half of people with schizophrenia die from tobacco-related diseases [93]. As such, it is imperative to consider their unique motivations for smoking and challenges in quitting when designing cessation initiatives.

1.4.2 Alcohol Use

Comorbid alcohol use is associated with poor clinical outcomes among people with schizophrenia. These include shorter duration of antipsychotic medication use, more medication discontinuations and missed pills, and higher rates of hospitalization and use of emergency services [102, 103]. Furthermore, those who use alcohol generally obtain less services overall. For example, veterans diagnosed with schizophrenia who used alcohol reported less use of services that promote clinical and functional recovery (e.g., general medical, mental health, occupational, and housing services) at the Veteran's Health Administration than those with schizophrenia who did not use alcohol [104]. The stigma associated with schizophrenia might be one reason for elevated rates of alcohol use as well as difficulty quitting. Higher levels of perceived stigma are associated with alcohol use disorder among people experiencing a FEP [105], and support groups such as Alcoholics Anonymous are underutilized among individuals with co-occurring psychotic disorders [106]. The unique needs of this population might better be met in dual-focused recovery groups such as Dual Recovery Anonymous [106].

1.4.3 Cannabis Use

The relationship between cannabis use and psychosis is multifaceted and complex. Cannabis users are at increased risk of developing psychosis, and this relationship appears to be dose dependent, so that heavy users are at a greater risk than light users [90]. Higher-potency cannabis with more concentrated Δ-9-tetrahydrocannabinol (THC) appears to be more harmful than lower potency [107]. However, there is preliminary evidence that another compound found in marijuana, cannabidiol (CBD), has therapeutic properties on its own and mitigates the harmful effects of THC [107]. Any lifetime cannabis use is associated with a 40% increase in risk of developing psychosis, and cannabis dependence is associated with a 240% increase [90]. Cannabis users have a two- to three-year earlier onset of illness than nonusers [90].

Research has overwhelmingly established a correlation between cannabis use and psychosis; however, the question of causation is still debated [108]. There are three potential explanations for the observed relationships: (1) Cannabis use triggers schizophrenia in individuals who would not have developed the illness had they not used the drug; (2) individuals with a predisposition to schizophrenia use cannabis to mitigate the prodromal symptoms of the disorder; and (3) there is a common cause such as childhood trauma or genetics that explains both cannabis use and the development of psychosis [108].

Additionally, there are negative impacts of cannabis use among people already diagnosed with psychotic disorders. Among this population, cannabis use is associated with poorer prognosis, including more pronounced positive symptoms, greater impairment in overall functioning, decreased medication adherence, more frequent relapse, and increased number of hospitalizations [90, 102, 109]. Discontinuing use reduces this risk of poor outcomes to that of never-users [90]. However, efforts to address cannabis use in early intervention treatment have been disappointing [110]. Future interventions should be designed to treat both schizophrenia-spectrum and substance use disorders together.

There are important limitations to consider when reviewing research on the relationship between cannabis use and schizophrenia, in particular an overrepresentation of men in Western countries as research participants. Rates, cultural acceptability, and legality of substance use differ across cultures as well as within cultures over time. Sex and gender may influence both genetic and cultural considerations. Thus, future research should consider these factors [108]. In addition, cannabis and tobacco are frequently used in combination, so it is difficult to decouple their effects in research on either one [108].

1.5 Suicide Risk

People with schizophrenia are at increased risk for suicide. The lifetime risk of suicide among people with schizophrenia is 5%, and the proportion of people with schizophrenia who attempt suicide is estimated to range from 25% to 50% [111]. This represents a 50- to 100-fold increase in suicidality compared to the general population [111]. People with schizophrenia tend to die by suicide at younger ages than those in the general population as well as those with other psychiatric disorders [112]. Considering these statistics, the issue of suicide among people with schizophrenia warrants attention and intervention in both clinical and nonclinical settings.

There are several important risk factors for suicide to consider among this population. In general, substance abuse increases the risk for suicide among people with and without schizophrenia [112, 113]. Among people with schizophrenia, a history of tobacco or alcohol use is associated with suicide attempts and completed suicide [111]. Comorbid depression is also associated with both suicidal ideation and suicide attempts in this population [111]. Suicidal ideation is higher among people who have more severe psychotic symptoms and a higher number of psychiatric hospitalizations [112, 113]. Suicide risk is correlated with timing around hospitalizations, with one-third of suicides among inpatients occurring during admission or within 1 week after discharge [112]. This risk is especially great if the reason for admission was a suicide attempt [112]. In general, previous suicide attempts are a significant risk factor for suicide, and people with schizophrenia who have previously attempted suicide have approximately three times greater risk of dying by suicide than those with no prior attempts [112].

Insight into illness, described in psychiatry as being able to recognize one's own mental illness and its consequences, impacts risk for suicide in people with schizophrenia in complicated ways [112]. It is suggested that greater insight is associated with increased risk of hopelessness, depression, and suicide [112]. However, greater insight is also generally associated with greater treatment adherence, a protective factor against suicide [112]. It may be that both patients with poor and good insight attempt suicide; those with poor insight may do so under the influence of psychotic symptoms and command hallucinations, while patients with good insight may do so under feelings of stress, shame, and stigma associated with schizophrenia [113].

1.6 Housing and Schizophrenia

Finding and maintaining suitable housing is often a challenge for people with schizophrenia. Since deinstitutionalization, many people with chronic mental illnesses live with family members [79]. However, living independently is associated with greater quality of life among people with schizophrenia [114], especially for those living in individualistic Western cultures such as the United States. In addition, a sizable percentage of people with schizophrenia are unstably housed. Among Clinical Antipsychotic Trials of Intervention Effectiveness (CATIE) participants, a representative sample of adults with schizophrenia seeking treatment in the United States, approximately 14% were unstably housed [79]. This means that they were unhoused or stayed in any given housing arrangement for less than 25 of the past 30 days [79]. An estimated 11% of unhoused people have schizophrenia compared to just 1% of the general population [77, 115]. Among people with SMI, those with schizophrenia are more likely to be unhoused than those with bipolar disorder and major depression [62].

A person's housing situation majorly impacts their ability to adequately manage mental illness. Only half of unhoused people with schizophrenia receive treatment [115]. Housing status is an independent risk factor for diminished functional capacity, such that unhoused people with schizophrenia-spectrum disorders performed worse than housed people, even though there were no significant differences between the groups in demographic, clinical, or neuropsychological tests [116]. This relationship between housing and mental status can create a devastating spiral. First, schizophrenia is a risk factor for becoming unhoused, and then, being unhoused leads to more psychiatric hospitalizations and further diminished functional capacity [78, 116].

It is important to consider finding and sustaining suitable housing arrangements a fundamental goal of comprehensive treatment for schizophrenia. One promising approach, Housing First, provides housing that is not contingent upon compliance with any treatment or abstinence from substances [117]. In this approach to treatment, housing is viewed as a human right and a necessary first step to obtaining and adhering to treatment. A study evaluating Housing First found that those who were placed in market rental accommodations with assertive community treatment significantly improved medication adherence compared to those randomized to treatment as usual and congregate Housing First [118]. Another study found the Housing First approach associated with significantly fewer inpatient days and decreased healthcare and residential costs [119].

1.7 Employment and Schizophrenia

The ability to work is understood to be a central issue in a person's life. Employment is part of almost every definition of recovery for those with mental illness [120]. Employment is associated with positive outcomes in social functioning, symptom levels, quality of life, and self-esteem [121]. It provides coping strategies and supports the process of recovery [120]. However, employment rates are low among this population, with only about 15% of CATIE study participants being competitively employed [122]. Another 13% participated in noncompetitive employment, but the majority (73%) were involved in no employment activities [122, 123]. Moreover, people with schizophrenia who are employed tend to make a low hourly wage and work substantially fewer hours than the general population [123] and frequently have brief job tenure [124].

Barriers to employment include stigmatization of mental illness, economic disincentives including the threat of losing benefits including medical insurance coverage, and an unmet need for support services to assist in finding and maintaining employment [121]. More severe positive symptoms and, to a lesser extent, negative symptoms are associated with poorer work outcomes [123]. Experiential negative symptoms, especially avolition or apathy, are related to job obtainment, hours worked, and wages earned [125].

Supported employment has been shown to have a positive effect on competitive job placement and job tenure; however, overall labor market conditions such as employment rates in the general population, access to welfare benefits, and availability of vocational services also influence employment opportunities and outcomes for people with schizophrenia [126]. Those who receive early intervention services are more likely to achieve good longitudinal employment outcomes over 10 years than those who receive standard care [127]. Improvements in social functioning after beginning treatment are also associated with future employment [128]. In addition to job-specific skills, people with schizophrenia who want to work need training for practical abilities such as work-related social skills, coping skills, and problem-solving skills [124].

1.8 Social Isolation and Loneliness

Social isolation and loneliness are important to consider among people with schizophrenia. People diagnosed with a schizophrenia-spectrum disorder report feeling lonelier than those without this type of disorder [129]. These feelings are reported to be widespread among this population. In an Australian national survey of people with psychosis, about 80% reported feeling lonely and 40% indicated that social isolation and loneliness were the top challenges in their lives [130]. The relationship between social isolation and schizophrenia is likely bidirectional. On the one hand, experiencing loneliness or social isolation is associated with poor mental health effects, and on the other, having a mental illness is associated with greater loneliness and social isolation. For example, a recent study showed that loneliness in a general population sample was associated with increased odds of psychotic experiences, a risk factor for developing schizophrenia or another mental illness later in life [131]. Among people with psychotic disorders, the perception that mental illness makes it hard to maintain close relationships and a fear of stigma or discrimination due to mental illness have been identified as the main barriers to social engagement [130].

Social isolation has many ill-health effects including early mortality [132–134]. Among people with schizophrenia, loneliness predicts comorbid illnesses such as substance use disorders, hypertension, and elevated hemoglobin A1c [129]. It has also been shown to be associated with increased care utilization, including visits to general practitioners, emergency department visits, and inpatient hospitalizations among people with psychotic disorders [135]. Socially isolated and lonely people are more than twice as likely to be "frequent users" of healthcare services compared to non-lonely people [135]. Importantly, higher levels of loneliness are significantly associated with suicidal behavior among people with psychotic disorders [136].

1.9 Stigma

Mental illness stigma is important to consider as it relates to schizophrenia. Link and Phelan [137] define stigma as a social phenomenon defined by four components: (1) It is fundamentally a label for an out-group; (2) the labeled differences are negative; (3) the differences separate "us" from "them"; and (4) the label and separation lead to status loss and discrimination. Social psychologists view stigma surrounding mental illness as consisting of three components: stereotypes, prejudice, and discrimination [138]. Stereotypes are cognitive representations depicting mentally ill people as possessing certain traits, prejudice involves negative affective states toward people with mental illnesses, and discrimination consists of negative behaviors or actions directed toward people with mental illnesses [138].

Schizophrenia stigma is evidenced by stereotypes depicting people with schizophrenia as dangerous, violent, at fault for their own illnesses, and unable to achieve most life goals, such as living and working independently [139]. These stereotypes lead to negative feelings against people with schizophrenia, which can in turn cause people to discriminate against them, such as by denying them a rental or falsely accusing them of a crime [138]. These stigmatized beliefs are especially relevant for someone who goes on to develop schizophrenia or a related disorder, as the possibility of devaluation and discrimination becomes personally relevant [140].

Individuals with schizophrenia have multiple intersecting identities which could lead to stigmatization and discrimination [141]. Double-disadvantage theory describes an accumulation of disadvantage with an increasing number of stigmatized identities [141]. For example, a Black man with schizophrenia who is unhoused, has a criminal background, and did not finish high school will likely experience considerably more stigma than a White woman with schizophrenia who has a college degree, is employed, and lives with family. Thus, the ways mental illness stigma intersects with other identities should be considered.

Schizophrenia is one of the most stigmatized mental illnesses, including among mental health professionals [142]. While mental health professionals are less likely than the general population to desire social distance from people with schizophrenia and perceive them as dangerous, they are more pessimistic about prognosis and schizophrenia outcomes [142]. They tend to hold a more biological view of the illness and have more positive beliefs about pharmacological treatment than the general population [142]. Biological beliefs about the etiology of schizophrenia lead to more negative attitudes such as exhibiting less empathy and more dehumanization [143, 144].

Beliefs about the etiology of mental illnesses have been extensively studied and used as a trigger point in anti-stigma efforts [145]. Specifically, this approach strongly emphasized the endorsement of biological and genetic causes of mental illness by explicitly portraying mental disorders as medical conditions that should be treated with medical treatments (e.g., "mental illness is an illness like any other") [145, 146]. This was intended to reduce attributions of responsibility and guilt toward people with mental illnesses by casting the cause of the illness as outside of their control [146]. However, this approach did not have the intended effect. Instead, it resulted in higher levels of negative stigma, including increased desire for social distance, prognostic pessimism, and higher perceptions of dangerousness [147, 148]. Evidence suggests that biogenetic illness models do not destigmatize mental illness and can actually worsen stigma [147]. Rather, interventions that provide education about mental illness and contact with people diagnosed with mental illnesses are more promising [149], especially if they are recovery-focused instead of symptom-focused [150].

1.10 Disparities in Schizophrenia Diagnosis

One of the longest-standing and most reproduced findings regarding the social epidemiology of schizophrenia is that it occurs more frequently among those of the lowest social class in society [151]. This finding spans countries and cultures [151]. One famous study conducted in 1958 showed that the poorest class was three times more likely than the wealthiest two classes to be treated for psychiatric problems, and the diagnosis with the strongest relationship with class was schizophrenia [152]. Those in the poorest class were eight times more likely than the wealthiest to be diagnosed with schizophrenia [152]. There are often put forth two explanations for this link between poverty and mental illness: social causation and social selection. The social causation hypothesis purports that growing up with the disadvantages and stress associated with poverty causes, at least in part, one to go on to develop psychosis or schizophrenia. Social selection explanations, on the other hand, suggest that people at all levels of income and class experience schizophrenia at the same rates, but those with the disorder are downwardly social mobile. Little evidence has supported the social selection hypothesis [153, 154]. It is important to note that social class exists along with other social locations and, as such, is heavily patterned by systems of racism, sexism, heterosexism, ageism, and ableism, creating increased risk of psychosis among many different marginalized groups [155].

Racial and ethnic disparities exist in the diagnosis of schizophrenia. A trend among international studies suggests that people who are immigrants and racial minorities are more likely to be diagnosed with a psychotic disorder than native citizens with a majority racial background [156]. Some even refer to migration and ethnicity as environmental risk factors for schizophrenia [157]. In the United States, Black and Latinx people are disproportionately diagnosed with psychotic disorders [156, 158]. Black people are diagnosed with schizophrenia at a rate three to four times greater than White people [156]. In fact, race was the strongest predictor of an admission diagnosis of schizophrenia in a study of people treated in state psychiatric hospitals [159]. Racial diagnostic bias, or clinicians making unwarranted judgments about people based on race, contributes to this documented disparity [156, 160]. Additionally, social and environmental conditions that affect psychosis risk (e.g., neighborhood factors, cumulative trauma and stress, and prenatal and perinatal complications) are also patterned by structural racism and inequality [161].

1.11 Summary

Despite its relatively low prevalence, schizophrenia presents a tremendous public health burden. People with the disorder face numerous challenges that greatly impact their mental and physical health. Stigmatized attitudes, beliefs, and behaviors drive many of these challenges. The drastically reduced life expectancy of this population brings attention to the fact that focused effort is needed to improve the health and well-being of people with schizophrenia. Innovative approaches to address the numerous problems in living associated with schizophrenia described here are urgently needed.

References

1. Levin BL, Petrila J, Hennessy KD. Mental health services: a public health perspective. 3rd ed. Oxford: Oxford University Press; 2010.
2. Gold JM. Cognitive deficits as treatment targets in schizophrenia. Schizophr Res. 2004;72(1):21–8.
3. Green MF, Horan WP, Lee J. Social cognition in schizophrenia. Nat Rev Neurosci. 2015;16(10):620.
4. Green MF, Horan WP, Lee J. Nonsocial and social cognition in schizophrenia: current evidence and future directions. World Psychiatry. 2019;18(2):146–61.

5. American Psychiatric Association. Diagnostic and statistical manual of mental disorders (DSM-5®). Washington, DC: American Psychiatric Publishing; 2013.
6. Galderisi S, Giordano GM. We are not ready to abandon the current schizophrenia construct, but should be prepared to do so. Schizophr Res. 2021;242:30.
7. Read J. Does 'schizophrenia' exist? Reliability and validity. In: Models of madness. London, UK: Routledge; 2013. p. 73–87.
8. Zwicker A, Denovan-Wright EM, Uher R. Gene–environment interplay in the etiology of psychosis. Psychol Med. 2018;48(12):1925–36.
9. Gottesman II, Laursen TM, Bertelsen A, Mortensen PB. Severe mental disorders in offspring with 2 psychiatrically ill parents. Arch Gen Psychiatry. 2010;67(3):252–7.
10. Joseph J. 'Schizophrenia' and heredity: why the emperor (still) has no genes. In: Models of madness. London, UK: Taylor & Francis; 2013. p. 72–89.
11. Susser ES, Lin SP. Schizophrenia after prenatal exposure to the Dutch Hunger Winter of 1944–1945. Arch Gen Psychiatry. 1992;49(12):983–8.
12. Nielsen PR, Meyer U, Mortensen PB. Individual and combined effects of maternal anemia and prenatal infection on risk for schizophrenia in offspring. Schizophr Res. 2016;172(1–3):35–40.
13. Attademo L, Bernardini F, Garinella R, Compton MT. Environmental pollution and risk of psychotic disorders: a review of the science to date. Schizophr Res. 2017;181:55–9.
14. Fineberg AM, Ellman LM, Schaefer CA, Maxwell SD, Shen L, Chaudhury NH, et al. Fetal exposure to maternal stress and risk for schizophrenia spectrum disorders among offspring: differential influences of fetal sex. Psychiatry Res. 2016;236:91–7.
15. Byrne M, Agerbo E, Bennedsen B, Eaton WW, Mortensen PB. Obstetric conditions and risk of first admission with schizophrenia: a Danish national register based study. Schizophr Res. 2007;97(1–3):51–9.
16. Mortensen PB, Pedersen CB, Westergaard T, Wohlfahrt J, Ewald H, Mors O, et al. Effects of family history and place and season of birth on the risk of schizophrenia. N Engl J Med. 1999;340(8):603–8.
17. Nosarti C, Reichenberg A, Murray RM, Cnattingius S, Lambe MP, Yin L, et al. Preterm birth and psychiatric disorders in young adult life. Arch Gen Psychiatry. 2012;69(6):610–7.
18. Trotta A, Di Forti M, Mondelli V, Dazzan P, Pariante C, David A, et al. Prevalence of bullying victimisation amongst first-episode psychosis patients and unaffected controls. Schizophr Res. 2013;150(1):169–75.
19. Varese F, Smeets F, Drukker M, Lieverse R, Lataster T, Viechtbauer W, et al. Childhood adversities increase the risk of psychosis: a meta-analysis of patient-control, prospective-and cross-sectional cohort studies. Schizophr Bull. 2012;38(4):661–71.
20. Marconi A, Di Forti M, Lewis CM, Murray RM, Vassos E. Meta-analysis of the association between the level of cannabis use and risk of psychosis. Schizophr Bull. 2016;42(5):1262–9.
21. Gurillo P, Jauhar S, Murray RM, MacCabe JH. Does tobacco use cause psychosis? Systematic review and meta-analysis. Lancet Psychiatry. 2015;2(8):718–25.
22. Fearon P, Kirkbride JB, Morgan C, Dazzan P, Morgan K, Lloyd T, et al. Incidence of schizophrenia and other psychoses in ethnic minority groups: results from the MRC AESOP Study. Psychol Med. 2006;36(11):1541–50.
23. Burns JK, Tomita A, Kapadia AS. Income inequality and schizophrenia: increased schizophrenia incidence in countries with high levels of income inequality. Int J Soc Psychiatry. 2014;60(2):185–96.
24. Agerbo E, Sullivan PF, Vilhjalmsson BJ, Pedersen CB, Mors O, Børglum AD, et al. Polygenic risk score, parental socioeconomic status, family history of psychiatric disorders, and the risk for schizophrenia: a Danish population-based study and meta-analysis. JAMA Psychiatry. 2015;72(7):635–41.
25. van Nierop M, Janssens M, Investigators GROoP, Bruggeman R, Cahn W, de Haan L, et al. Evidence that transition from health to psychotic disorder can be traced to semi-

ubiquitous environmental effects operating against background genetic risk. PLoS One. 2013;8(11):e76690.
26. Stepniak B, Papiol S, Hammer C, Ramin A, Everts S, Hennig L, et al. Accumulated environmental risk determining age at schizophrenia onset: a deep phenotyping-based study. Lancet Psychiatry. 2014;1(6):444–53.
27. O'Donoghue B, Lyne J, Madigan K, Lane A, Turner N, O'Callaghan E, et al. Environmental factors and the age at onset in first episode psychosis. Schizophr Res. 2015;168(1–2):106–12.
28. Mauritz MW, Goossens PJ, Draijer N, Van Achterberg T. Prevalence of interpersonal trauma exposure and trauma-related disorders in severe mental illness. Eur J Psychotraumatol. 2013;4(1):19985.
29. Cusack KJ, Grubaugh AL, Knapp RG, Frueh BC. Unrecognized trauma and PTSD among public mental health consumers with chronic and severe mental illness. Community Ment Health J. 2006;42(5):487–500.
30. Walsh K, McLaughlin KA, Hamilton A, Keyes KM. Trauma exposure, incident psychiatric disorders, and disorder transitions in a longitudinal population representative sample. J Psychiatr Res. 2017;92:212–8.
31. Read J, Goodman L, Morrison A, Ross C, Aderhold V. Childhood trauma, loss and stress. In: Models of madness: Psychological, social and biological approaches to schizophrenia. Brunner-Routledge: Hove, East Sussex, UK. 2004. p. 223–52.
32. Read J. Child abuse and severity of disturbance among adult psychiatric inpatients. Child Abuse Negl. 1998;22(5):359–68.
33. Kelleher I, Keeley H, Corcoran P, Ramsay H, Wasserman C, Carli V, et al. Childhood trauma and psychosis in a prospective cohort study: cause, effect, and directionality. Am J Psychiatr. 2013;170(7):734–41.
34. Janssen I, Krabbendam L, Bak M, Hanssen M, Vollebergh W, de Graaf R, et al. Childhood abuse as a risk factor for psychotic experiences. Acta Psychiatr Scand. 2004;109(1):38–45.
35. Neria Y, Bromet EJ, Sievers S, Lavelle J, Fochtmann LJ. Trauma exposure and posttraumatic stress disorder in psychosis: findings from a first-admission cohort. J Consult Clin Psychol. 2002;70(1):246.
36. Bendall S, Hulbert CA, Alvarez-Jimenez M, Allott K, McGorry PD, Jackson HJ. Testing a model of the relationship between childhood sexual abuse and psychosis in a first-episode psychosis group: the role of hallucinations and delusions, posttraumatic intrusions, and selective attention. J Nerv Ment Dis. 2013;201(11):941–7.
37. Van Dam D, Korver-Nieberg N, Velthorst E, Meijer C, De Haan L. Childhood maltreatment, adult attachment and psychotic symptomatology: a study in patients, siblings and controls. Soc Psychiatry Psychiatr Epidemiol. 2014;49(11):1759–67.
38. Goodman LA, Rosenberg SD, Mueser KT, Drake RE. Physical and sexual assault history in women with serious mental illness: prevalence, correlates, treatment, and future research directions. Schizophr Bull. 1997;23(4):685–96.
39. Cloitre M, Tardiff K, Marzuk PM, Leon AC, Portera L. Childhood abuse and subsequent sexual assault among female inpatients. J Trauma Stress. 1996;9(3):473–82.
40. Insel T, Cuthbert B, Garvey M, Heinssen R, Pine DS, Quinn K, et al. Research domain criteria (RDoC): toward a new classification framework for research on mental disorders. Am Psychiatric Assoc. 2010;167:748–51.
41. Frame L, Morrison AP. Causes of posttraumatic stress disorder in psychotic patients. Arch Gen Psychiatry. 2001;58(3):305–6.
42. Morrison AP, Frame L, Larkin W. Relationships between trauma and psychosis: a review and integration. Br J Clin Psychol. 2003;42(4):331–53.
43. Tarrier N, Khan S, Cater J, Picken A. The subjective consequences of suffering a first episode psychosis: trauma and suicide behaviour. Soc Psychiatry Psychiatr Epidemiol. 2007;42(1):29–35.
44. Jarvis GE. The social causes of psychosis in North American psychiatry: a review of a disappearing literature. Can J Psychiatry. 2007;52(5):287–94.

45. Read J, Bentall RP, Fosse R. Time to abandon the bio-bio-bio model of psychosis: exploring the epigenetic and psychological mechanisms by which adverse life events lead to psychotic symptoms. Epidemiol Psychiatr Sci. 2009;18(4):299–310.
46. Deacon BJ. The biomedical model of mental disorder: a critical analysis of its validity, utility, and effects on psychotherapy research. Clin Psychol Rev. 2013;33(7):846–61.
47. Thompson N. Mental health and well-being: alternatives to the medical model. New York, NY: Routledge; 2019.
48. Center for Behavioral Health Statistics and Quality. 2017 national survey on drug use and health: detailed tables. In: Administration SAaMHS, editor. Rockville, 2018.
49. Kessler RC, Aguilar-Gaxiola S, Alonso J, Chatterji S, Lee S, Ormel J, et al. The global burden of mental disorders: an update from the WHO World Mental Health (WMH) surveys. Epidemiol Psychiatr Sci. 2009;18(1):23–33.
50. Seabury SA, Axeen S, Pauley G, Tysinger B, Schlosser D, Hernandez JB, et al. Measuring the lifetime costs of serious mental illness and the mitigating effects of educational attainment. Health Aff. 2019;38(4):652–9.
51. de Mooij LD, Kikkert M, Theunissen J, Beekman ATF, de Haan L, Duurkoop PWRA, et al. Dying too soon: excess mortality in severe mental illness. Front Psych. 2019;10(855) https://doi.org/10.3389/fpsyt.2019.00855.
52. Fagiolini A, Goracci A. The effects of undertreated chronic medical illnesses in patients with severe mental disorders. J Clin Psychiatry. 2009;70:22.
53. Chang C-K, Hayes RD, Perera G, Broadbent MT, Fernandes AC, Lee WE, et al. Life expectancy at birth for people with serious mental illness and other major disorders from a secondary mental health care case register in London. PLoS One. 2011;6(5):e19590.
54. Walker ER, McGee RE, Druss BG. Mortality in mental disorders and global disease burden implications: a systematic review and meta-analysis. JAMA Psychiatry. 2015;72(4):334–41.
55. Luciano A, Meara E. Employment status of people with mental illness: national survey data from 2009 and 2010. Psychiatr Serv. 2014;65(10):1201–9.
56. Frank RG, Koss C. Mental health and labor markets productivity loss and restoration, Disease Control Priorities Project. Geneva: World Health Organization; 2005.
57. Baldwin ML, Marcus SC. Labor market outcomes of persons with mental disorders. Ind Relat J Econ Soc. 2007;46(3):481–510.
58. Kessler RC, Heeringa S, Lakoma MD, Petukhova M, Rupp AE, Schoenbaum M, et al. Individual and societal effects of mental disorders on earnings in the United States: results from the national comorbidity survey replication. Am J Psychiatr. 2008;165(6):703–11.
59. Burnett-Zeigler I, Ilgen MA, Bohnert K, Miller E, Islam K, Zivin K. The impact of psychiatric disorders on employment: results from a national survey (NESARC). Community Ment Health J. 2013;49(3):303–10.
60. Mechanic D, Bilder S, McAlpine DD. Employing persons with serious mental illness. Health Aff. 2002;21(5):242–53.
61. Glasheen C, Forman-Hoffman VL, Hedden S, Ridenour TA, Wang J, Porter JD. Residential transience among adults: prevalence, characteristics, and association with mental illness and mental health service use. Community Ment Health J. 2019;55(5):784–97.
62. Folsom DP, Hawthorne W, Lindamer L, Gilmer T, Bailey A, Golshan S, et al. Prevalence and risk factors for homelessness and utilization of mental health services among 10,340 patients with serious mental illness in a large public mental health system. Am J Psychiatr. 2005;162(2):370–6.
63. Smartt C, Prince M, Frissa S, Eaton J, Fekadu A, Hanlon C. Homelessness and severe mental illness in low-and middle-income countries: scoping review. BJPsych Open. 2019;5(4)
64. Childress S, Reitzel LR, Maria DS, Kendzor DE, Moisiuc A, Businelle MS. Mental illness and substance use problems in relation to homelessness onset. Am J Health Behav. 2015;39(4):549–55.
65. Teplin LA. Criminalizing mental disorder: the comparative arrest rate of the mentally ill. Am Psychol. 1984;39(7):794.

66. Teplin LA. Keeping the peace: police discretion and mentally ill persons. Natl Inst Justice J. 2000;244:8–15.
67. Al-Rousan T, Rubenstein L, Sieleni B, Deol H, Wallace RB. Inside the nation's largest mental health institution: a prevalence study in a state prison system. BMC Public Health. 2017;17(1):1–9.
68. Fazel S, Hayes AJ, Bartellas K, Clerici M, Trestman R. Mental health of prisoners: prevalence, adverse outcomes, and interventions. Lancet Psychiatry. 2016;3(9):871–81.
69. Steadman HJ, Osher FC, Robbins PC, Case B, Samuels S. Prevalence of serious mental illness among jail inmates. Psychiatr Serv. 2009;60(6):761–5.
70. Bradley-Engen MS, Cuddeback GS, Gayman MD, Morrissey JP, Mancuso D. Trends in state prison admission of offenders with serious mental illness. Psychiatr Serv. 2010;61(12):1263–5.
71. Morrissey J, Meyer P, Cuddeback G. Extending assertive community treatment to criminal justice settings: origins, current evidence, and future directions. Community Ment Health J. 2007;43(5):527–44.
72. Charlson FJ, Ferrari AJ, Santomauro DF, Diminic S, Stockings E, Scott JG, et al. Global epidemiology and burden of schizophrenia: findings from the global burden of disease study 2016. Schizophr Bull. 2018;44(6):1195–203.
73. Chong HY, Teoh SL, Wu DB-C, Kotirum S, Chiou C-F, Chaiyakunapruk N. Global economic burden of schizophrenia: a systematic review. Neuropsychiatr Dis Treat. 2016;12:357.
74. Millier A, Schmidt U, Angermeyer M, Chauhan D, Murthy V, Toumi M, et al. Humanistic burden in schizophrenia: a literature review. J Psychiatr Res. 2014;54:85–93.
75. Vos T, Abajobir AA, Abate KH, Abbafati C, Abbas KM, Abd-Allah F, et al. Global, regional, and national incidence, prevalence, and years lived with disability for 328 diseases and injuries for 195 countries, 1990–2016: a systematic analysis for the Global Burden of Disease Study 2016. Lancet (London, England). 2017;390(10100):1211–59. https://doi.org/10.1016/s0140-6736(17)32154-2.
76. World Health Organization. The global burden of disease: 2004 update. Geneva: World Health Organization; 2008.
77. Ayano G, Tesfaw G, Shumet S. The prevalence of schizophrenia and other psychotic disorders among homeless people: a systematic review and meta-analysis. BMC Psychiatry. 2019;19(1):1–14.
78. Foster A, Gable J, Buckley J. Homelessness in schizophrenia. Psychiatr Clin. 2012;35(3):717–34.
79. Tsai J, Stroup TS, Rosenheck RA. Housing arrangements among a national sample of adults with chronic schizophrenia living in the United States: a descriptive study. J Community Psychol. 2011;39(1):76–88.
80. Hall D, Lee L-W, Manseau MW, Pope L, Watson AC, Compton MT. Major mental illness as a risk factor for incarceration. Psychiatr Serv. 2019;70(12):1088–93.
81. Azad MC, Shoesmith WD, Al Mamun M, Abdullah AF, Naing DKS, Phanindranath M, et al. Cardiovascular diseases among patients with schizophrenia. Asian J Psychiatr. 2016;19:28–36.
82. Ringen PA, Engh JA, Birkenaes AB, Dieset I, Andreassen OA. Increased mortality in schizophrenia due to cardiovascular disease – a non-systematic review of epidemiology, possible causes, and interventions. Front Psych. 2014;5:137.
83. Drope J, Liber AC, Cahn Z, Stoklosa M, Kennedy R, Douglas CE, et al. Who's still smoking? Disparities in adult cigarette smoking prevalence in the United States. CA Cancer J Clin. 2018;68(2):106–15.
84. Jakobsen AS, Speyer H, Nørgaard HCB, Karlsen M, Hjorthøj C, Krogh J, et al. Dietary patterns and physical activity in people with schizophrenia and increased waist circumference. Schizophr Res. 2018;199:109–15.
85. Davidson S, Judd F, Jolley D, Hocking B, Thompson S, Hyland B. Cardiovascular risk factors for people with mental illness. Aust N Z J Psychiatry. 2001;35(2):196–202.

86. Hunt GE, Large MM, Cleary M, Lai HMX, Saunders JB. Prevalence of comorbid substance use in schizophrenia spectrum disorders in community and clinical settings, 1990–2017: systematic review and meta-analysis. Drug Alcohol Depend. 2018;191:234–58.
87. Dixon L. Dual diagnosis of substance abuse in schizophrenia: prevalence and impact on outcomes. Schizophr Res. 1999;35:S93–S100.
88. Hartz SM, Pato CN, Medeiros H, Cavazos-Rehg P, Sobell JL, Knowles JA, et al. Comorbidity of severe psychotic disorders with measures of substance use. JAMA Psychiatry. 2014;71(3):248–54.
89. Hjorthøj C, Fohlmann A, Nordentoft M. Treatment of cannabis use disorders in people with schizophrenia spectrum disorders – a systematic review. Addict Behav. 2009;34(6–7):520–5.
90. Hasan A, von Keller R, Friemel CM, Hall W, Schneider M, Koethe D, et al. Cannabis use and psychosis: a review of reviews. Eur Arch Psychiatry Clin Neurosci. 2020;270(4):403–12.
91. Bhalla IP, Stefanovics EA, Rosenheck RA. Clinical epidemiology of single versus multiple substance use disorders: polysubstance use disorder. Med Care. 2017;55:S24–32.
92. Carney R, Yung A, Amminger GP, Bradshaw T, Glozier N, Hermens DF, et al. Substance use in youth at risk for psychosis. Schizophr Res. 2017;181:23–9.
93. Callaghan RC, Veldhuizen S, Jeysingh T, Orlan C, Graham C, Kakouris G, et al. Patterns of tobacco-related mortality among individuals diagnosed with schizophrenia, bipolar disorder, or depression. J Psychiatr Res. 2014;48(1):102–10.
94. Castillo-Sánchez M, Fàbregas-Escurriola M, Bergè-Baquero D, Fernández-SanMartín MI, Goday-Arno A. Screening of cardiovascular risk factors in patients with schizophrenia and patients treated with antipsychotic drugs: are we equally exhaustive as with the general population? Clin Exp Hypertens. 2017;39(5):441–7.
95. Ayerbe L, Forgnone I, Foguet-Boreu Q, González E, Addo J, Ayis S. Disparities in the management of cardiovascular risk factors in patients with psychiatric disorders: a systematic review and meta-analysis. Psychol Med. 2018;48(16):2693–701.
96. Hickling LM, Perez-Iglesias R, de la Foz VO-G, Balanzá-Martínez V, McGuire P, Crespo-Facorro B, et al. Tobacco smoking and its association with cognition in first episode psychosis patients. Schizophr Res. 2018;192:269–73.
97. Cather C, Hoeppner S, Pachas G, Pratt S, Achtyes E, Cieslak KM, et al. Improved depressive symptoms in adults with schizophrenia during a smoking cessation attempt with varenicline and behavioral therapy. J Dual Diagn. 2017;13(3):168–78.
98. Ahmed S, Virani S, Kotapati VP, Bachu R, Adnan M, Khan AM, et al. Efficacy and safety of varenicline for smoking cessation in schizophrenia: a meta-analysis. Front Psych. 2018;9:428.
99. Travaglini LE, Li L, Brown CH, Bennett ME. Predictors of smoking cessation group treatment engagement among veterans with serious mental illness. Addict Behav. 2017;75:103–7.
100. Sagud M, Peles AM, Pivac N. Smoking in schizophrenia: recent findings about an old problem. Curr Opin Psychiatry. 2019;32(5):402–8.
101. Burda K, Czubak A, Nowakowska E, Kus K, Metelska J, Nowakowska A. Interactions of nicotine and drugs used in the treatment of mental illnesses with respect to cognitive functions. Arzneimittelforschung. 2010;60(09):527–43.
102. Oluwoye O, Monroe-DeVita M, Burduli E, Chwastiak L, McPherson S, McClellan JM, et al. Impact of tobacco, alcohol and cannabis use on treatment outcomes among patients experiencing first episode psychosis: data from the national RAISE-ETP study. Early Interv Psychiatry. 2019;13(1):142–6.
103. Ahn S, Choi Y, Choi W, Jo YT, Kim H, Lee J, et al. Effects of comorbid alcohol use disorder on the clinical outcomes of first-episode schizophrenia: a nationwide population-based study. Ann General Psychiatry. 2021;20(1):1–8.
104. Pedersen ER, Huang W, Cohen AN, Young AS. Alcohol use and service utilization among veterans in treatment for schizophrenia. Psychol Serv. 2018;15(1):21.
105. Brunette MF, Mueser KT, Babbin S, Meyer-Kalos P, Rosenheck R, Correll CU, et al. Demographic and clinical correlates of substance use disorders in first episode psychosis. Schizophr Res. 2018;194:4–12.

106. Archibald L, Brunette MF, Wallin DJ, Green AI. Alcohol use disorder and schizophrenia or schizoaffective disorder. Alcohol Res Curr Rev. 2019;40(1):arcr.v40.1.06.
107. Colizzi M, Ruggeri M, Bhattacharyya S. Unraveling the intoxicating and therapeutic effects of cannabis ingredients on psychosis and cognition. Front Psychol. 2020;11:833.
108. Hamilton I, Monaghan M. Cannabis and psychosis: are we any closer to understanding the relationship? Curr Psychiatry Rep. 2019;21(7):1–4.
109. Patel RS, Sreeram V, Vadukapuram R, Baweja R. Do cannabis use disorders increase medication non-compliance in schizophrenia?: United States Nationwide inpatient cross-sectional study. Schizophr Res. 2020;224:40–4.
110. McDonell MG, Oluwoye O. Cannabis use in first episode psychosis: what we have tried and why it hasn't worked. BMC Med. 2019;17(1):1–2.
111. Cassidy RM, Yang F, Kapczinski F, Passos IC. Risk factors for suicidality in patients with schizophrenia: a systematic review, meta-analysis, and meta-regression of 96 studies. Schizophr Bull. 2018;44(4):787–97.
112. Hettige NC, Bani-Fatemi A, Sakinofsky I, De Luca V. A biopsychosocial evaluation of the risk for suicide in schizophrenia. CNS Spectr. 2018;23(4):253–63.
113. De Sousa A, Shah B, Shrivastava A. Suicide and schizophrenia: an interplay of factors. Curr Psychiatry Rep. 2020;22(12):1–5.
114. Hansson L, Middelboe T, Sørgaard K, Bengtsson-Tops A, Bjarnason O, Merinder L, et al. Living situation, subjective quality of life and social network among individuals with schizophrenia living in community settings. Acta Psychiatr Scand. 2002;106(5):343–50.
115. Folsom D, Jeste DV. Schizophrenia in homeless persons: a systematic review of the literature. Acta Psychiatr Scand. 2002;105(6):404–13.
116. Stergiopoulos V, Burra T, Rourke S, Hwang S. Housing status as an independent predictor of functional capacity in patients with schizophrenia. J Nerv Ment Dis. 2011;199(11):854–60.
117. Baxter AJ, Tweed EJ, Katikireddi SV, Thomson H. Effects of Housing First approaches on health and well-being of adults who are homeless or at risk of homelessness: systematic review and meta-analysis of randomised controlled trials. J Epidemiol Community Health. 2019;73(5):379–87.
118. Rezansoff SN, Moniruzzaman A, Fazel S, McCandless L, Procyshyn R, Somers JM. Housing first improves adherence to antipsychotic medication among formerly homeless adults with schizophrenia: results of a randomized controlled trial. Schizophr Bull. 2017;43(4):852–61.
119. Tinland A, Loubière S, Boucekine M, Boyer L, Fond G, Girard V, et al. Effectiveness of a housing support team intervention with a recovery-oriented approach on hospital and emergency department use by homeless people with severe mental illness: a randomised controlled trial. Epidemiol Psychiatr Sci. 2020;29
120. Schennach R, Musil R, Möller H-J, Riedel M. Functional outcomes in schizophrenia: employment status as a metric of treatment outcome. Curr Psychiatry Rep. 2012;14(3):229–36.
121. Marwaha S, Johnson S. Schizophrenia and employment. Soc Psychiatry Psychiatr Epidemiol. 2004;39(5):337–49.
122. Rosenheck R, Leslie D, Keefe R, McEvoy J, Swartz M, Perkins D, et al. Barriers to employment for people with schizophrenia. Am J Psychiatr. 2006;163(3):411–7.
123. Salkever DS, Karakus MC, Slade EP, Harding CM, Hough RL, Rosenheck RA, et al. Measures and predictors of community-based employment and earnings of persons with schizophrenia in a multisite study. Psychiatr Serv. 2007;58(3):315–24.
124. Carmona VR, Gómez-Benito J, Rojo-Rodes JE. Employment support needs of people with schizophrenia: a scoping study. J Occup Rehabil. 2019;29(1):1–10.
125. Llerena K, Reddy LF, Kern RS. The role of experiential and expressive negative symptoms on job obtainment and work outcome in individuals with schizophrenia. Schizophr Res. 2018;192:148–53.
126. Carmona VR, Gómez-Benito J, Huedo-Medina TB, Rojo JE. Employment outcomes for people with schizophrenia spectrum disorder: a meta-analysis of randomized controlled trials. Int J Occup Med Environ Health. 2017;30(3):345.

127. Chan SKW, Pang HH, Yan KK, Hui CLM, Suen YN, Chang WC, et al. Ten-year employment patterns of patients with first-episode schizophrenia-spectrum disorders: comparison of early intervention and standard care services. Br J Psychiatry. 2020;217(3):491–7.
128. Hasegawa T, Hashimoto T, Kanahara N, Yamanaka H, Ishige M, Sato Y, et al. Identifying improvable employment-related factors in schizophrenia patients. Psychiatry Res. 2018;266:199–205.
129. Tremeau F, Antonius D, Malaspina D, Goff DC, Javitt DC. Loneliness in schizophrenia and its possible correlates. An exploratory study. Psychiatry Res. 2016;246:211–7. https://doi.org/10.1016/j.psychres.2016.09.043.
130. Stain HJ, Galletly CA, Clark S, Wilson J, Killen EA, Anthes L, et al. Understanding the social costs of psychosis: the experience of adults affected by psychosis identified within the second Australian National Survey of psychosis. Aust N Z J Psychiatry. 2012;46(9):879–89.
131. Narita Z, Stickley A, DeVylder J. Loneliness and psychotic experiences in a general population sample. Schizophr Res. 2020;218:146–50. https://doi.org/10.1016/j.schres.2020.01.018.
132. Holt-Lunstad J, Smith TB, Baker M, Harris T, Stephenson D. Loneliness and social isolation as risk factors for mortality: a meta-analytic review. Perspect Psychol Sci. 2015;10(2):227–37.
133. Holt-Lunstad J, Smith TB, Layton JB. Social relationships and mortality risk: a meta-analytic review. PLoS Med. 2010;7(7):e1000316.
134. House JS, Landis KR, Umberson D. Social relationships and health. Science. 1988;241(4865):540–5.
135. Badcock JC, Di Prinzio P, Waterreus A, Neil AL, Morgan VA. Loneliness and its association with health service utilization in people with a psychotic disorder. Schizophr Res. 2020;223:105–11. https://doi.org/10.1016/j.schres.2020.05.059.
136. Badcock JC, Di Prinzio P, Ambrosi T, Waterreus A, Morgan VA. Loneliness, social isolation and suicide risk in people with psychotic disorders. Schizophr Res. 2021;233:60–1. https://doi.org/10.1016/j.schres.2021.06.037.
137. Link BG, Phelan JC. Conceptualizing stigma. Annu Rev Sociol. 2001;27:363–85.
138. Ottati V, Bodenhausen GV, Newman LS. Social psychological models of mental illness stigma. In: On the stigma of mental illness: practical strategies for research and social change. Washington, DC: American Psychological Association; 2005. p. 99–128.
139. Angermeyer MC, Dietrich S. Public beliefs about and attitudes towards people with mental illness: a review of population studies. Acta Psychiatr Scand. 2006;113(3):163–79.
140. Link BG, Phelan JC. Labeling and stigma. In: Handbook of the sociology of mental health. Dordrecht: Springer; 2013. p. 525–41.
141. Oexle N, Corrigan PW. Understanding mental illness stigma toward persons with multiple stigmatized conditions: implications of intersectionality theory. Psychiatr Serv. 2018;69(5):587–9.
142. Valery K-M, Prouteau A. Schizophrenia stigma in mental health professionals and associated factors: a systematic review. Psychiatry Res. 2020;290:113068.
143. Lebowitz MS, W-k A. Effects of biological explanations for mental disorders on clinicians' empathy. Proc Natl Acad Sci. 2014;111(50):17786–90.
144. Pavon G, Vaes J. Bio-genetic vs. psycho-environmental conceptions of schizophrenia and their role in perceiving patients in human terms. Psychosis. 2017;9(3):245–53.
145. Mannarini S, Rossi A. Assessing mental illness stigma: a complex issue. Front Psychol. 2019;9:2722.
146. Corrigan PW. Mental health stigma as social attribution: implications for research methods and attitude change. Clin Psychol Sci Pract. 2000;7(1):48.
147. Angermeyer MC, Holzinger A, Carta MG, Schomerus G. Biogenetic explanations and public acceptance of mental illness: systematic review of population studies. Br J Psychiatry. 2011;199(5):367–72.
148. Kvaale EP, Haslam N, Gottdiener WH. The 'side effects' of medicalization: a meta-analytic review of how biogenetic explanations affect stigma. Clin Psychol Rev. 2013;33(6):782–94.

149. Morgan AJ, Reavley NJ, Ross A, San Too L, Jorm AF. Interventions to reduce stigma towards people with severe mental illness: systematic review and meta-analysis. J Psychiatr Res. 2018;103:120–33.
150. Norman RM, Li Y, Sorrentino R, Hampson E, Ye Y. The differential effects of a focus on symptoms versus recovery in reducing stigma of schizophrenia. Soc Psychiatry Psychiatr Epidemiol. 2017;52(11):1385–94.
151. Kohn ML. The interaction of social class and other factors in the etiology of schizophrenia. Am J Psychiatry. 1976;
152. Hollingshead AB, Redlich FC. Social class and mental illness: community study. 1958.
153. Fox JW. Social class, mental illness, and social mobility: the social selection-drift hypothesis for serious mental illness. J Health Soc Behav. 1990;31:344–53.
154. Hudson CG. Socioeconomic status and mental illness: tests of the social causation and selection hypotheses. Am J Orthopsychiatry. 2005;75(1):3–18.
155. Brown LS. The great divide: trauma and social class. In: Brown LS, editor. Cultural competence in trauma therapy: beyond the flashback. American Psychological Association; 2008. p. 197–213. https://doi.org/10.1037/11752-010.
156. Schwartz RC, Blankenship DM. Racial disparities in psychotic disorder diagnosis: a review of empirical literature. World J Psychiatry. 2014;4(4):133.
157. Dean K, Murray RM. Environmental risk factors for psychosis. Dialogues Clin Neurosci. 2005;7(1):69.
158. Hamilton JE, Heads AM, Meyer TD, Desai PV, Okusaga OO, Cho RY. Ethnic differences in the diagnosis of schizophrenia and mood disorders during admission to an academic safety-net psychiatric hospital. Psychiatry Res. 2018;267:160–7.
159. Barnes A. Race and hospital diagnoses of schizophrenia and mood disorders. Soc Work. 2008;53(1):77–83.
160. Schwartz EK, Docherty NM, Najolia GM, Cohen AS. Exploring the racial diagnostic bias of schizophrenia using behavioral and clinical-based measures. J Abnorm Psychol. 2019;128(3):263.
161. Anglin DM, Ereshefsky S, Klaunig MJ, Bridgwater MA, Niendam TA, Ellman LM, et al. From womb to neighborhood: a racial analysis of social determinants of psychosis in the United States. Am J Psychiatr. 2021;178(7):599–610.
162. Hjorthøj C, Stürup AE, McGrath JJ, Nordentoft M. Years of potential life lost and life expectancy in schizophrenia: a systematic review and meta-analysis. The Lancet Psychiatry. 2017;4(4):295–301.

Chapter 2
Current Approaches to Schizophrenia Treatment

2.1 Goals of Treatment: Remission and Recovery

Recovery in schizophrenia is possible and should be a central goal of treatment. While early conceptualizations of schizophrenia hypothesized it to be progressive and irreversible, contemporary evidence does not support this assertion. End states of the disorder range from severe cases requiring multiple hospitalizations to cases in which a single illness episode is followed by complete remission of symptoms [1, 2]. Despite this, treatment goals set by clinicians tend to be modest, focusing on achieving remission by controlling symptoms and behavior and attaining stability [1]. Historically, less attention has been paid to the more complex concept of recovery [1].

Remission is a clinical state of symptom reduction [1]. In 2005, the Remission in Schizophrenia Working Group published operationalized criteria for remission based on severity and duration [3]. These criteria dictate that a person in remission has at most a mild symptom intensity that does not influence their behavior for 6 months [1, 3]. Remission can be achieved through maintenance treatment with antipsychotic medication [3]. Personal factors associated with increased probability of remission have been identified as better premorbid functioning, milder symptoms at baseline, early response to treatment, and shorter duration of untreated psychosis [3]. According to this working group, remission is a necessary but not sufficient step toward recovery [1]. Most people who experience a first episode of psychosis achieve clinical remission within the first year of treatment [4].

Recovery, on the other hand, is a much more complex phenomenon. Definitions of recovery can be based on personal goals and aspirations [5]. Leamy and colleagues define it as "psychological recovery from consequences of the illness" [6]. Their conceptualization includes the following processes: finding hope, reestablishment of identity, finding meaning in life, and taking responsibility for recovery [6]. The Substance Abuse and Mental Health Services Administration (SAMHSA) has

M. Evans, *Peer Support Services Reaching People with Schizophrenia*, https://doi.org/10.1007/978-3-031-29042-8_2

defined recovery as "a process of change through which individuals improve their health and wellness, live a self-directed life, and strive to reach their full potential" [7]. They put forth four dimensions of recovery: health, home, purpose, and community [7]. In another perspective, the CHIME framework, five recovery processes are proposed: connectedness, hope and optimism about the future, identity, meaning in life, and empowerment [5]. Recovery is generally thought of as a process and not an outcome [8].

Another distinction in defining recovery warrants attention: that between *recovery from* mental illness and *recovery in* mental illness [9]. Recovery from mental illness, or clinical recovery, is conceptualized as a process through which people with mental illnesses regain functional capabilities and experience remission from signs and symptoms [9]. This term is more easily defined and measured than recovery in mental illness and is, thus, frequently used in clinical practice and research [9]. On the other hand, recovery in mental illness, or personal recovery, is a process through which individuals with mental illness live their lives and pursue their goals and aspirations, with dignity and autonomy, while also living with symptoms of mental illness or vulnerability to relapse [9]. The focus is on one's strengths and remaining capabilities to live a full life despite mental illness [9]. This conceptualization of *recovery in*, while not referred to as such, is the objective of most noncommunicable disease management. For example, in diabetes, the goal is not to eradicate the illness but rather successfully manage it with diet, exercise, and medication. These definitions and distinctions are important when considering approaches to treatment.

2.2 Pharmacological Treatment

In general, the first line of treatment recommended for those with schizophrenia is prescription of antipsychotic medication [10]. Antipsychotic medications are placed into two different categories: first-generation antipsychotics (FGAs) and second-generation antipsychotics (SGAs). Developed in the 1950s, FGAs work by blocking the dopamine D-2 receptors [10, 11]. They have been shown to be effective in reducing positive symptoms but ineffective at mitigating negative symptoms [12]. Significant side effects of FGAs include extrapyramidal symptoms such as tremors, slurred speech, akathisia, dystonia, and tardive dyskinesia [12].

First introduced in the 1980s, SGAs act as dopamine agonists and have replaced FGAs as the schizophrenia treatment of choice [12]. They have been proven effective in treating positive symptoms, but there is considerable debate as to whether they are efficacious in the reduction of negative symptoms [12]. In a systematic review of the efficacy of antipsychotic medication in treating negative symptoms, only one drug, amisulpride, was identified as outperforming placebo [13]. While SGAs were developed to improve on the shortcomings of FGAs, they also have significant adverse side effects [12]. These include sedation, hypotension, weight gain, and sexual dysfunction [12]. SGAs are also associated with increased cardiometabolic risk, including elevated lipids and the development of type 2 diabetes mellitus [11, 12]. While it is recommended that all patients treated with antipsychotic medications are monitored closely for cardiometabolic risk factors, the monitoring of physical health parameters among people with schizophrenia tends to be poor [11].

Efficacy of antipsychotic medications varies according to the stage of illness, with those experiencing the first episode of psychosis responding faster and better to antipsychotics than those at later stages [10]. The largest effect of antipsychotic medications takes place within the first week of taking it [11]. If a patient does not respond to an antipsychotic treatment within 4–6 weeks, it is recommended to switch to another with a different receptor-binding profile [11]. Approximately 30% of people diagnosed with schizophrenia meet the criteria for treatment resistance, defined as symptoms that do not respond to two different antipsychotic medications at therapeutic doses and for a duration of 6–8 weeks [11]. Studies have found few differences in effectiveness between the two generations of medications among people with treatment-resistant schizophrenia [11, 12]. Only one drug, clozapine, has shown effectiveness in treatment-resistant schizophrenia; however, it carries a heavy burden of adverse reactions, such as sedation and significant weight gain [11].

Medication nonadherence is common in any chronic illness, and rates of nonadherence are higher among people with schizophrenia than among people with other chronic illnesses [11]. In this population, rates of medication nonadherence have been estimated to be between 50% and 75% [11, 14–16]. Medication discontinuation or nonadherence can occur due to intolerable side effects, the persistence of residual positive symptoms, and poor therapeutic alliance [11]. Furthermore, side effects, stigma, relationships with other people, economic issues, fear and coercion have all been identified as factors influencing adherence or non-adherence with medication [17]. Prescription of antipsychotic medication comprises an important part of the management of schizophrenia; however, continued adherence needs to be considered. Furthermore, antipsychotic medications do not singularly treat all symptoms, and they often produce debilitating side effects.

2.3 Psychosocial Treatment

Antipsychotic medications are likely to work better in conjunction with some form of psychosocial treatment. Several psychosocial treatments frequently used in the treatment of schizophrenia include cognitive behavioral therapy, cognitive remediation therapy, cognitive adaptation training, psychoeducation, family interventions, social skills training, and supported employment [18, 19]. These treatments and their documented benefits are briefly described below. Also described are two approaches to organizing treatment, early intervention programs for treating first-episode psychosis and assertive community treatment.

Cognitive behavioral therapy (CBT) is a highly structured and standardized therapy that intends to help patients with schizophrenia cope with psychotic symptoms by examining and reevaluating their thoughts and perceptions [18]. In this approach, the therapist accepts the patient's perspective of reality and determines how to use it to assist the patient in appropriately managing their life problems [18]. Cognitive behavioral therapy has been shown to be associated with improved functional outcomes, improved quality of life, and reduced relapse and positive symptoms [18, 19].

Cognitive remediation therapy aims to enhance executive functioning and social cognition through information restructuring or reorganization, effective use of environmental aids and probes, and a wide range of techniques concerning cognitive functioning [18]. Cognitive remediation techniques can be deployed on computers or by paper and pencil [19]. This approach is associated with improvement in cognitive functioning and social behaviors [18].

Cognitive adaptation training employs environmental supports to target severe functional impairments associated with psychosis, including techniques such as labeling and utilization of signs and alarms in an individual's environment to encourage activities of daily living, self-care, and medication management [19]. It is generally undertaken on a weekly basis for a period of 9 months and has been found to be associated with an increase in global functioning and a reduction in relapse [19].

Psychoeducation focuses on providing information about the illness, its treatment, behavior management, problem-solving, coping skills, and access to community mental health services [18]. It is generally led by health professionals [18] and is intended to increase knowledge and understanding of the illness, decrease self-stigmatization, and promote treatment engagement [19]. Psychoeducation has been shown to be associated with an increase in global functioning, a decrease in relapse rates, and a reduction of positive symptoms [18, 19].

Family intervention approaches can be directed at family members alone, without the involvement of the person with schizophrenia, or involve the person and their family as a unit. These approaches tend to focus on family dynamics and interactions, such as expressed emotion, in an aim to help the family better support their loved one who has schizophrenia [18]. Family interventions may promote the use of problem-solving, communication, coping, or illness management skills [19]. They generally consist of at least 10 sessions over a six-month period and have been shown to be effective at preventing relapse as well as associated with improvement in positive symptoms [18, 19].

Social skills training consists of three main components: receiving skills (social perception), processing skills (social cognition), and sending information skills (behavioral responding or expression) [18]. To target these elements of social competence, it employs techniques such as role modeling, positive reinforcement, and behavioral rehearsals [19]. Social skills training generally lasts between 5 and 6 months and is intended to improve social functioning and increase social support [19]. Compared to treatment as usual, it has been shown to be associated with increases in global functioning and improvements in core illness symptoms, including negative symptoms [19]. It has also been shown to be associated with moderate improvements in interpersonal skills and community functioning [18].

Supported employment assists individuals in finding competitive employment, supports them in that employment, and teaches them skills and strategies to maintain employment [19]. Also known as the Individual Placement and Support (IPS) model, this approach involves weekly support for both the client and employer during the first month on the job [19]. After that, support for the client is provided monthly throughout the first 12 months of employment [19]. This approach is associated with better employment outcomes, including higher rates of employment, more hours worked, longer duration of employment, and greater earnings [19].

Early intervention for first-episode psychosis (FEP) services includes a range of interventions to help identify and treat individuals experiencing FEP [19]. Interventions are delivered by a multidisciplinary team and include psychopharmacological treatment, family education, psychosocial interventions (e.g., psychoeducation, CBT, vocational interventions), and peer support [19]. The aim of this approach is to reduce the clinical and psychosocial declines related to the onset of a psychotic disorder [19]. Individuals generally attend FEP services weekly for a period of 2 years [19]. This approach is associated with improvement in global functioning and quality of life as well as with a reduced likelihood of relapse [19]. Individuals in FEP programs are also more likely to be working or in school than those receiving treatment as usual [19].

Finally, another approach to organizing treatment, assertive community treatment (ACT), focuses on persistent, intensive outreach among those with high use of inpatient services, a history of poor engagement with services which has led to frequent relapse and/or social breakdown, or who need immediate assistance in a crisis [18]. These treatment teams are characterized by very low staff-to-patient ratios, high frequency of contacts, and the provision of comprehensive and multidisciplinary care with 24-hour availability [18]. The multidisciplinary care team consists of roles such as psychiatric care providers, nurses, employment specialists, co-occurring substance use disorder specialists, and peer specialists [19]. ACT has been shown to substantially reduce psychiatric hospitalizations, increase housing stability, increase employment, and moderately improve positive symptoms and quality of life [18–20].

2.4 Treatment Engagement

Despite the many options available, many people with schizophrenia are not engaging with treatment fully or at all. There are numerous factors that affect whether people engage with and benefit from schizophrenia treatment. In a nationally representative cross-sectional survey, the National Comorbidity Survey Replication (NCS-R), it was estimated that approximately half of people with SMI received no treatment in the year prior to the survey and one-sixth of people who began treatment discontinued prematurely within that year [21]. Taken together, this means that only approximately 35% of people with SMI in this study received stable treatment [21]. Furthermore, only 15% received minimally adequate treatment, defined as receiving a prescription for an appropriate medication and attending four or more mental health visits or attending eight or more mental health visits without receipt of a prescription [22]. There are certain populations that are more difficult to engage in care, including those experiencing an FEP and those with dual diagnoses of mental illness and substance use disorders [23].

Disengagement with care is associated with poorer outcomes, including symptom exacerbations, hospitalizations, and being unhoused [24–26]. Dropping out of treatment or missing appointments is associated with poorer outcomes and increased risk of relapse [27]. In a comprehensive study in the US, patients who kept a follow-up appointment had a 10% chance of being rehospitalized within a year, whereas for those who did not keep an appointment, the chances of being rehospitalized were 25% [27].

Reasons for disengaging with care vary and include both psychosocial and structural barriers to care. The most common reason cited in the NCS-R for dropping out of treatment was a desire to solve the problem on one's own [21]. A large proportion of respondents in this study believed that mental health treatment was not effective, and this belief was associated with an increased likelihood of dropping out of treatment [28]. Additionally, feeling uncomfortable in mental health treatment, a likely proxy for perceived stigma, was associated with higher rates of dropout [28]. Attitudinal and evaluative barriers (e.g., perceived ineffectiveness of treatment, negative experiences with providers, stigma) have been shown to be more important in deciding to discontinue mental health treatment than structural barriers [29]. Stigma is an important factor to consider in engagement with mental health care, with people reporting they avoid or drop out of care because they do not want to be labeled, have experienced judgment or disrespect from providers, or feel shame or embarrassment about their mental illness [30]. As such, people report being uncomfortable talking to mental health providers as a barrier to receiving treatment [30].

The perspectives of patients and providers regarding reasons for disengagement from treatment do not necessarily align [31]. In a qualitative study investigating reasons for treatment disengagement, clients reported that disengagement occurred because the services failed to meet their needs and they experienced difficulties with the treatment relationship and trust, while providers viewed disengagement as due to a lack of insight, difficulties coping with their illness, lack of family support for engaging in care, and logistical barriers [31]. This discrepancy in perspectives may be due in part to provider stigma, and interventions that promote continued treatment engagement for people with schizophrenia are needed.

2.5 Racial and Ethnic Disparities in Schizophrenia Treatment

Racism and mental illness stigma intersect to produce disparities in the ways schizophrenia treatment is provided. Black people are more likely to be hospitalized when they seek care for schizophrenia than are White people [32, 33]. People with SMI from racial and ethnic minority groups are more likely to be admitted to psychiatric emergency services than community support services [34]. Furthermore, Black people with SMI are more likely than White people to be involuntarily hospitalized, to use crisis services, and to enter emergency treatment by means of law enforcement [35–38]. Black people receive higher doses of antipsychotic medications, increased use of depot medication, and are less likely to receive second-generation antipsychotics, which are associated with less severe side effects, than White people [39, 40]. Racial and ethnic minorities experience poorer outcomes when they do receive treatment and are at higher risk for disengagement from treatment [41]. It is estimated that Black people with SMI are five times less likely to receive minimally adequate care than are White people [22].

Research has found that these documented disparities in mental health treatment widen at moderate and serious levels of psychological distress compared to no or mild levels of distress, while the opposite is true for physical health disparities [42]. This suggests that these disparities are not primarily driven by overuse by people of the majority race (e.g., the so-called "worried well" users with little or no mental health problems) but rather indicate problems in meeting the needs of minoritized people with significant mental health issues [42]. Furthermore, these disparities did not alleviate with access to health insurance provided by the Affordable Care Act [43]. Increased efforts to remedy these injustices are warranted.

2.6 Summary

Current approaches to schizophrenia treatment include prescription of antipsychotic medication and a variety of psychosocial treatments. However, evidenced by the immense degree of disability and disenfranchisement experienced by people with schizophrenia, current treatments are not adequately ameliorating the damaging effects of the disorder and its consequences. There remains an unmet need in schizophrenia treatment to achieve personal recovery and improve functional status, in addition to remission of positive symptoms. Thus, additional complementary approaches to standard treatment should be explored and evaluated for their potential to promote positive outcomes among people with schizophrenia. One innovative complementary approach is the provision of holistic peer support.

References

1. Emsley R, Chiliza B, Asmal L, Lehloenya K. The concepts of remission and recovery in schizophrenia. Curr Opin Psychiatry. 2011;24(2):114–21.
2. Zipursky RB. Why are the outcomes in patients with schizophrenia so poor? J Clin Psychiatry. 2014;75(suppl 2):22442.
3. AlAqeel B, Margolese HC. Remission in schizophrenia: critical and systematic review. Harv Rev Psychiatry. 2013;20(6):281–97.

4. Zipursky RB, Reilly TJ, Murray RM. The myth of schizophrenia as a progressive brain disease. Schizophr Bull. 2013;39(6):1363–72.
5. Leamy M, Bird V, Le Boutillier C, Williams J, Slade M. Conceptual framework for personal recovery in mental health: systematic review and narrative synthesis. Br J Psychiatry. 2011;199(6):445–52.
6. Andresen R, Oades L, Caputi P. The experience of recovery from schizophrenia: towards an empirically validated stage model. Aust N Z J Psychiatry. 2003;37(5):586–94.
7. Substance Abuse and Mental Health Services Administration: SAMHSA's working definition of recovery. https://store.samhsa.gov/sites/default/files/d7/priv/pep12-recdef.pdf (2012). Accessed 3 Dec 2021.
8. Frese FJ, Davis WW. The consumer–survivor movement, recovery, and consumer professionals. Prof Psychol Res Pract. 1997;28(3):243.
9. Davidson L, Roe D. Recovery from versus recovery in serious mental illness: one strategy for lessening confusion plaguing recovery. J Ment Health. 2007;16(4):459–70.
10. Chien WT, Yip AL. Current approaches to treatments for schizophrenia spectrum disorders, part I: an overview and medical treatments. Neuropsychiatr Dis Treat. 2013;9:1311.
11. Lally J, MacCabe JH. Antipsychotic medication in schizophrenia: a review. Br Med Bull. 2015;114(1):169–79.
12. Abou-Setta AM, Mousavi SS, Spooner C, Schouten JR, Pasichnyk D, Armijo-Olivo S, et al. First-generation versus second-generation antipsychotics in adults: comparative effectiveness. 2012.
13. Krause M, Zhu Y, Huhn M, Schneider-Thoma J, Bighelli I, Nikolakopoulou A, et al. Antipsychotic drugs for patients with schizophrenia and predominant or prominent negative symptoms: a systematic review and meta-analysis. Eur Arch Psychiatry Clin Neurosci. 2018;268(7):625–39.
14. Velligan D, Weiden P, Sajatovic M, Scott J, Carpenter D, Ross R, et al. Expert Consensus Panel on Adherence Problems in Serious and Persistent Mental Illness. The expert consensus guideline series: adherence problems in patients with serious and persistent mental illness. J Clin Psychiatry. 2009;70(suppl 4):1–46.
15. Lacro JP, Dunn LB, Dolder CR, Jeste DV. Prevalence of and risk factors for medication nonadherence in patients with schizophrenia: a comprehensive review of recent literature. J Clin Psychiatry. 2002;63(10):892–909.
16. Gilmer TP, Dolder CR, Lacro JP, Folsom DP, Lindamer L, Garcia P, et al. Adherence to treatment with antipsychotic medication and health care costs among Medicaid beneficiaries with schizophrenia. Am J Psychiatr. 2004;161(4):692–9.
17. Wade M, Tai S, Awenat Y, Haddock G. A systematic review of service-user reasons for adherence and nonadherence to neuroleptic medication in psychosis. Clin Psychol Rev. 2017;51:75–95.
18. Chien WT, Leung SF, Yeung FK, Wong WK. Current approaches to treatments for schizophrenia spectrum disorders, part II: psychosocial interventions and patient-focused perspectives in psychiatric care. Neuropsychiatr Dis Treat. 2013;9:1463.
19. McDonagh MS, Dana T, Kopelovich SL, Monroe-DeVita M, Blazina I, Bougatsos C, et al. Psychosocial interventions for adults with schizophrenia: an overview and update of systematic reviews. Psychiatric Services. 2022;73(3):299–312. https://doi.org/10.1176/appi.ps.202000649.
20. Clarke GN, Herinckx HA, Kinney RF, Paulson RI, Cutler DL, Lewis K, et al. Psychiatric hospitalizations, arrests, emergency room visits, and homelessness of clients with serious and persistent mental illness: findings from a randomized trial of two ACT programs vs. usual care. Ment Health Serv Res. 2000;2(3):155–64.
21. Kessler RC, Berglund PA, Bruce ML, Koch JR, Laska EM, Leaf PJ, et al. The prevalence and correlates of untreated serious mental illness. Health Serv Res. 2001;36(6 Pt 1):987.
22. Wang PS, Demler O, Kessler RC. Adequacy of treatment for serious mental illness in the United States. Am J Public Health. 2002;92(1):92–8.

23. Dixon LB, Holoshitz Y, Nossel I. Treatment engagement of individuals experiencing mental illness: review and update. World Psychiatry. 2016;15(1):13–20.
24. Fischer EP, McCarthy JF, Ignacio RV, Blow FC, Barry KL, Hudson TJ, et al. Longitudinal patterns of health system retention among veterans with schizophrenia or bipolar disorder. Community Ment Health J. 2008;44(5):321–30.
25. Kreyenbuhl J, Nossel IR, Dixon LB. Disengagement from mental health treatment among individuals with schizophrenia and strategies for facilitating connections to care: a review of the literature. Schizophr Bull. 2009;35(4):696–703.
26. O'Brien A, Fahmy R, Singh SP. Disengagement from mental health services. Soc Psychiatry Psychiatr Epidemiol. 2009;44(7):558–68.
27. Nelson EA, Maruish ME, Axler JL. Effects of discharge planning and compliance with outpatient appointments on readmission rates. Psychiatr Serv. 2000;51(7):885–9.
28. Edlund MJ, Wang PS, Berglund PA, Katz SJ, Lin E, Kessler RC. Dropping out of mental health treatment: patterns and predictors among epidemiological survey respondents in the United States and Ontario. Am J Psychiatr. 2002;159(5):845–51.
29. Mojtabai R, Olfson M, Sampson NA, Jin R, Druss B, Wang PS, et al. Barriers to mental health treatment: results from the National Comorbidity Survey Replication. Psychol Med. 2011;41(8):1751–61.
30. Clement S, Schauman O, Graham T, Maggioni F, Evans-Lacko S, Bezborodovs N, et al. What is the impact of mental health-related stigma on help-seeking? A systematic review of quantitative and qualitative studies. Psychol Med. 2015;45(1):11–27.
31. Smith TE, Easter A, Pollock M, Pope LG, Wisdom JP. Disengagement from care: perspectives of individuals with serious mental illness and of service providers. Psychiatr Serv. 2013;64(8):770–5.
32. Durbin A, Rudoler D, Durbin J, Laporte A, Callaghan RC. Examining patient race and area predictors of inpatient admission for schizophrenia among hospital users in California. J Immigr Minor Health. 2014;16(6):1025–34.
33. Rost K, Hsieh Y-P, Xu S, Menachemi N, Young AS. Potential disparities in the management of schizophrenia in the United States. Psychiatr Serv. 2011;62(6):613–8.
34. Young AS, Chinman MJ, Cradock-O'Leary JA, Sullivan G, Murata D, Mintz J, et al. Characteristics of individuals with severe mental illness who use emergency services. Community Ment Health J. 2005;41(2):159–68.
35. Atdjian S, Vega WA. Disparities in mental health treatment in US racial and ethnic minority groups: implications for psychiatrists. Psychiatr Serv. 2005;56(12):1600–2.
36. Barnes A. Race, schizophrenia, and admission to state psychiatric hospitals. Adm Policy Ment Health Ment Health Serv Res. 2004;31(3):241–52.
37. Snowden LR. Barriers to effective mental health services for African Americans. Ment Health Serv Res. 2001;3(4):181–7.
38. Snowden LR, Pingitore D. Frequency and scope of mental health service delivery to African Americans in primary care. Ment Health Serv Res. 2002;4(3):123–30.
39. Kreyenbuhl J, Zito JM, Buchanan RW, Soeken KL, Lehman AF. Racial disparity in the pharmacological management of schizophrenia. Schizophr Bull. 2003;29(2):183–94.
40. Kuno E, Rothbard AB. Racial disparities in antipsychotic prescription patterns for patients with schizophrenia. Am J Psychiatr. 2002;159(4):567–72.
41. Maura J, de Mamani AW. Mental health disparities, treatment engagement, and attrition among racial/ethnic minorities with severe mental illness: a review. J Clin Psychol Med Settings. 2017;24(3):187–210.
42. Biener AI, Zuvekas SH. Do racial and ethnic disparities in mental health treatment vary with underlying mental health? Med Care Res Rev. 2021;78(4):392–403. https://doi.org/10.1177/1077558720903589.
43. Creedon TB, Cook BL. Access to mental health care increased but not for substance use, while disparities remain. Health Aff. 2016;35(6):1017–21.

Chapter 3
Theoretical Foundations of Peer Support

The theoretical bases of peer support are varied and come from several disciplines including public health, psychology, and sociology. While there is no single theory of peer support, understanding the theoretical underpinnings of the practice is important to aid understanding of the associated benefits and challenges. This chapter outlines several of the broad theoretical perspectives informing peer support work, provides a perspective which defines peer support by function rather than form, and concludes with the presentation of a conceptual model of peer support services that reach people with schizophrenia and related disorders.

3.1 Social Relationships and Social Support

Fundamentally, peer support interventions are based on evidence of the salubrious effects of social support. People who have strong social ties live longer and have better mental and physical health than their socially isolated counterparts [1–6], while social isolation and loneliness are associated with poorer mental and physical health [7, 8]. Social ties are thought to promote health in large part through the provision of social support, or the functional content of relationships. Social support is associated with increased health-promoting behaviors, including medication adherence [9–11], smoking cessation [12, 13], and weight loss [14, 15]. In addition to physical health benefits, high levels of social support have been shown to be associated with better mental health [4, 16]. The documented effects of social ties are hypothesized to work through different pathways [17]. Directly, supportive ties may influence an individual's health and well-being by meeting basic human needs for companionship, intimacy, and a sense of belonging [18]. Indirectly, social ties and social support may affect health by assisting individuals in accessing coping resources as well as influencing the frequency and duration of their exposure to stressors [17].

M. Evans, *Peer Support Services Reaching People with Schizophrenia*,
https://doi.org/10.1007/978-3-031-29042-8_3

Social support is often classified as comprising the categories emotional, instrumental, informational, and appraisal support [19]. Emotional support consists of expressions of empathy, love, trust, and caring [19]. Instrumental support comprises tangible aid and services, while informational support consists of advice, suggestions, and information [19]. Finally, appraisal support involves providing information that is useful for self-evaluation [19]. Peer supporters can provide each of these types of social support in a variety of ways.

While these types of support are conceptually distinct, they can be conveyed in an overlapping manner, often in the same interaction [20]. In peer support interventions, emotional support is pervasive and is often closely tied with informational, instrumental, and appraisal support. Anecdotally, people often state when first encountering peer support that they desire informational or instrumental support; however, over time emotional support increases as other support needs are met. In other words, that a peer supporter is available to fulfill informational and instrumental support needs lends itself to developing emotional support [20]. Emotional support can be conveyed even in the absence of explicit conversations about emotions. Rather, shared activities and sensitivity to informational and instrumental support needs are also ways of conveying emotional support. Additionally, the grounded nature of peer support often lends itself to the provision of instrumental support, as those who have similar lived experiences are more likely to know what might be helpful and accessible to their clients than providers of professional services. For example, while professionals may be able to provide referrals to social services, those with lived experience of navigating these complex systems are likely able to give much more concrete and helpful guidance.

One important distinction among types of social support is that between directive and nondirective support. Directive support is prescriptive and takes over responsibility for tasks and outcomes, while nondirective support is more accepting of receivers' preferences and feelings and cooperative with their plans. Peer support generally emphasizes nondirective support [21]. While patient-provider relationships are hierarchical in nature and, thus, tend to be directive, peer support relationships are nonhierarchical, and peers and clients work together to determine options and potential best courses of action for each individual client on their personal recovery journey [21]. However, there may be instances where directive support is warranted and more helpful than nondirective support, such as when facing acute stressors or situations in which people are unsure of what to do [22–25] or situations for which they lack coping skills [26]. In such cases, directive support may be especially enhanced by the peer supporter being familiar with the circumstances of the recipient and having a practical understanding of what may be helpful in these circumstances.

3.2 The Value of Experiential Knowledge and Expertise

Experiential knowledge, knowing about a topic as a subject rather than objectively, is a key aspect of most peer support interventions in mental health [27]. Medical knowledge and care are traditionally provided in a very top-down manner, with experts providing patients with knowledge and care from the vantage point of their extensive training being bestowed upon the patient. As it values lived experience expertise, or being an expert through lived experience, peer support fundamentally disrupts this model. The lived experience of living with mental illness and navigating services provides a unique point of view from which peer supporters operate. Unlike formalized objective knowledge, experiential knowledge allows the peer supporter to integrate their knowledge of mental illness with self-awareness and connect it to their own lifeworld [27].

In the field of mental health, a history of lived experience of mental illness or substance use is often a requirement of those employed as peer support workers. It is thought that this shared lived experience provides something unique beyond the concrete services offered by peer supporters. Thus, understanding how to best utilize experiential knowledge in peer support is an area of great interest and need. Additionally, what constitutes a shared lived experience may differ from person to person. For some, it may be sharing a specific diagnosis; for others, a specific experience, such as being hospitalized in a psychiatric inpatient setting or being unhoused; for still others, it may be a shared cultural identity. While acknowledging that mental illness and substance use frequently co-occur, an interesting aspect to the lived experience qualification is that the way it is applied may result in someone with a primary substance use disorder providing support to someone without a substance use disorder but a serious mental illness, or vice versa. Cultivating a deeper understanding of an optimal match between peers and those they support may advance the field.

3.3 Social Cognitive Theory and Observational Learning

Social cognitive theory, and especially its construct of observational learning, informs peer support. Developed by Albert Bandura and originally termed social learning theory, social cognitive theory emphasizes reciprocal determinism, the idea that individuals and their environments interact to produce behavior [28]. Thus, environments affect individuals, but additionally, individuals affect their environments. According to this theory, human behavior is the product of a dynamic interplay of individual, behavioral, and environmental factors [29]. Observational learning refers to the phenomenon of learning to perform new behaviors through media or interpersonal exposure [28]. Social cognitive theory posits that people are more likely to imitate the behavior of people they perceive to be similar to themselves [30]. Role modeling such as this is an especially important function of peer support programs, especially those organized around a shared lived experience as a basis for support. Observational learning would suggest that people experiencing mental health challenges are more likely to imitate the behavior of others who have similar experiences and, thus, peer supporters role modeling successful coping skills will support the genesis of these behaviors among their those they support.

3.4 Social Comparison Theory

In addition to social cognitive theory, peer support is informed by social comparison theory [31]. This theory purports that people have a need to evaluate themselves by comparing with others [31]. Upward social comparisons occur when the individual views the comparator as better off than themselves, which may provide hope and motivation to follow in their footsteps [31]. Downward social comparisons, on the other hand, occur when individuals view the comparators as worse off than themselves, resulting in their feeling better about their circumstances [31]. Both types of comparisons may be made in peer support work [32]. In some cases, peer workers might serve as role models and examples of what is possible in recovery, while in others, individuals with mental health challenges may recognize by comparisons with their peer support worker that other people with greater challenges have embarked on a recovery journey and perhaps their own challenges are also not insurmountable.

3.5 Stigma and Modified Labeling Theory

Stigma and Goffman's notion of the "total institution" [33] plays an important role in any discussion about people with serious mental illnesses. In his work *Asylums,* Goffman (1961) writes that people in mental hospitals and other total institutions are often identified by a singular role, such as mental patient, and this identity overshadows all other aspects of the person. This applies to people with schizophrenia, who are often viewed as little more than their diagnoses [34]. Furthermore, their actions are likely to be viewed as caused by and reflecting their illness, rather than justified by any other means [34]. For example, if a person diagnosed with schizophrenia does not adhere to or engage with treatment, providers are likely to attribute this to poor insight rather than consider that the treatment may be unacceptable to the patient for any number of valid reasons [35]. Culturally tailored peer support, on the other hand, may provide a more nuanced understanding informed by lived experience. Providing an escape, even if only temporary, from this singular devalued role of mental patient can be profoundly beneficial in helping the person to maintain a holistic identity that extends beyond mental illness.

Modified labeling theory postulates that people develop conceptions of mental illness early on in life as part of socialization and form expectations about the likelihood that a person with a mental illness will be rejected by significant others, including friends, employers, or intimate partners, or thought to be less trustworthy, intelligent, and competent [36]. These beliefs are especially relevant for a person who goes on to develop a mental illness, as the possibility of devaluation and discrimination becomes personally relevant [36]. To the extent that stigmatized beliefs become part of a person's worldview, this perception can have serious negative consequences, including more constricted social networks [36]. People who fear they will be stigmatized often withdraw from social interaction, resulting in a social network that often consists only of household members [36].

Stigma is not only an interpersonal phenomenon; rather, it operates at all levels of the socioecological model. Self-stigma occurs when a person internalizes mental illness stigma which leads them to feel shame and hopelessness [36]. Interpersonal stigma, enacted as well as perceived or threatened, leads people with mental illnesses to act less confidently and more defensively [36]. Additionally, people with mental illnesses who fear rejection tend to withdraw and have insular support networks consisting mainly of the people in their household [36]. Public stigma can lead to label avoidance, meaning someone avoids the unfair loss of status and opportunity that accompanies stigmatizing labels of mental illness by not seeking treatment, even if they themselves do not internalize such stigma [37]. Providers of mental health services are also prone to endorse stigmatized beliefs about mental illness, and this can affect how they interact with and treat patients [38].

3.6 Key Functions of Peer Support

Informed by extensive work with peer support programs around the world, Peers for Progress put forth five key functions of peer support [39–42]. While peer supporters may be known by different names in different contexts (e.g., community health workers, *promotoras,* peer support specialists, etc.), this conceptualization aims to define peer supporters by what they do, not what they are called. The five key functions of peer support put forth are as follows: (1) "being there," (2) assistance in self-management, (3) social and emotional support, (4) linkage to clinical care and community resources, and (5) ongoing support. Standardization by function, not content, provides a template or organizational framework for the adaptation of peer support models and programs to fit the unique needs of the population served. The five key functions are explained in detail below with a focus on how they are relevant to peer support for people with schizophrenia.

3.6.1 "Being there"

Providing human connection, or "just being there," is identified as a fundamental feature of peer support [43]. This personal connection facilitates the basis on which peer support services are provided and has been identified as important in and of itself. In many different languages and cultures, there is an equivalent saying to, "It wasn't anything she said or did, it was just knowing she was there" [26]. This expression of unconditional support may be more visible in less hierarchical and formal relationships (e.g., those between peer supporters and those they support) than in conventional provider-patient relationships. Other scholarship has coined other terms for similar constructs—common humanity [32] and holding space [44], for example. Lending support to its importance, a recent study showed benefits to older adults of just talking with college students who were trained to simply engage in conversation with those they support [45].

3.6.2 Assistance in Self-Management

Successfully managing one's mental health often requires close attention and daily action. Peer supporters can assist in these self-management tasks. For many individuals, understanding and implementing the care plans developed by mental healthcare providers can be daunting. Appointments are often brief and can involve numerous and potentially complicated treatment recommendations for the patient. Peer supporters can help individuals translate what care providers recommend into specific, actionable plans [40]. In other words, care providers may help people figure out *what to do*, while peer supporters help them to figure out *how to do it*. Additionally, they can help to identify barriers to effective self-management and devise ways to address them. Peers can draw from their lived experience in making these plans, which tends to convey more credibility than advice from professionals. Furthermore, assistance in daily self-management of mental health problems includes activities such as psychoeducation and various types of skills training, including social skills. Peer supporters can assist people to solve problems and overcome social and emotional barriers to sustaining evidence-based self-management behaviors [46].

3.6.3 Social and Emotional Support

Maintaining motivation for self-management of mental illness is not an easy task, and support and encouragement are often needed. Peer supporters can provide an opportunity for the client to share emotional and feeling states [40]. Emotional support may help individuals to cope with the reality of being diagnosed with schizophrenia or a related disorder and the considerable distress that may accompany it. Furthermore, instrumental, informational, and appraisal support are also provided by peer supporters in accordance with a person's needs.

3.6.4 Linkage to Clinical Care and Community Resources

Peer supporters can help patients recognize when they should access health care or community resources and facilitate the timely linkage to services [47]. Beyond simple linkage to mental health services, evidence shows that peer support is also associated with greater trust in and rapport with treatment providers and an increased willingness to take an active role in their own treatment [48, 49]. Additionally, peer supporters can share knowledge of other community resources that might be beneficial to those they support as they navigate not only dealing with mental illness but also the stresses and problems associated with daily life. These resources may include heathcare services, behavioral health services, community-based programs, financial resources, and social services.

3.6.5 Ongoing Support

Peer support is ideally extended over time and is not a time-limited intervention. Although using peers to teach time-limited courses [50] or to promote preventive services such as screenings and immunizations [51] can be effective, oftentimes the focus of a peer is to support and encourage the ongoing behaviors and lifestyle factors that contribute to healthy living for the rest of an individual's life. Like many chronic illnesses, schizophrenia tends to have a long course with significant needs over time. Ongoing support is needed to help people effectively manage the disorder and live full and satisfying lives. Sustained relationships and ongoing support can confer benefits throughout the different stages of illness and life course.

3.7 A Socioecological Model of Peer Support Reaching People with Schizophrenia

Built upon a socioecological framework, a general conceptual model illustrating the features and multilevel inputs and outcomes of peer support is presented in Fig. 3.1. Socioecological models emphasize that individuals are nested within interpersonal, organizational, community, and policy environments, and interventions should focus on changes at more than one level if they are to be effective [52]. Reciprocal determinism, a key feature of socioecological models, suggests that changes at one level impact changes at other levels [52]. While peer support interventions may at first seem to be mainly operating on the interpersonal level, this conceptual model identifies inputs and outputs at each level of the socioecological model.

Peer support as an intervention is influenced heavily by policy support, such as Medicaid reimbursement for peer support specialist services. Additionally, many peer support programs are community based, benefitting from community support and high levels of social capital. At the organizational level, mental health services and community resources provide the infrastructure and needed resources to facilitate the operation of peer support services. Inclusion of peer supporters on mental healthcare teams is another example of an organizational level input, as is clear role definition for peer supporters and differentiation of that role from other members of the care team. Interpersonally, peer support inputs include role modeling and

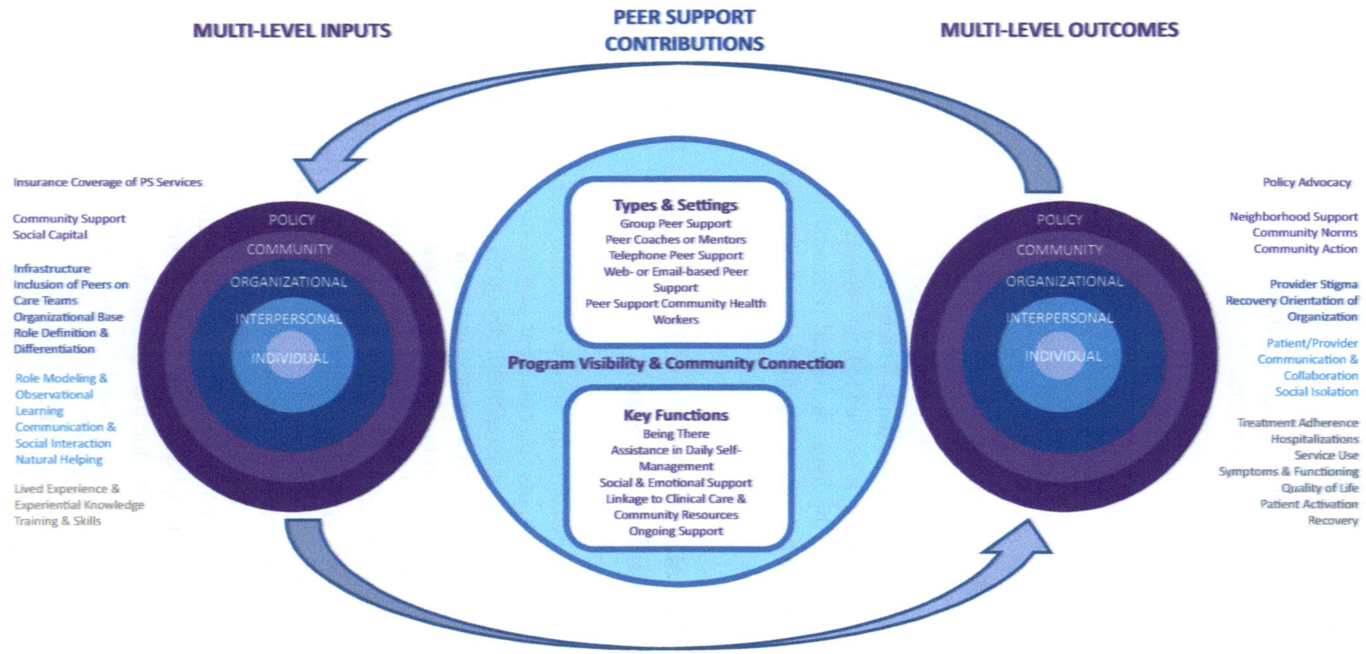

Fig. 3.1 Conceptual model of peer support

observational learning, communication and social interactions, and natural helping. Each individual peer supporter brings their unique lived experience and experiential knowledge, as well as their training and skills.

These multilevel inputs support the development and operation of peer support programs. Adherence to the core features of peer support, the five key functions of peer support described above, allow for adaptation of peer support interventions so that they can be provided in a variety of different forms and settings. For example, peer support can be provided in face-to-face group meetings, one-to-one by peer coaches or mentors, via telephone, or online. Beyond the functions and settings of peer support, the visibility of the program and its connections in the community can invoke change among people not directly impacted by or involved with peer support. The simple fact that peer support programs exist and are active in the community can help to challenge stigma about the role of people with mental illnesses in society and influence community norms about mental health, illness, and recovery.

The provision of peer support can also have impacts at all levels of the socioecological model. By putting faces to the experience of living with mental illness, peer support can mobilize policy advocacy efforts and effect policy change. By being visible and providing needed services in the community, peer supporters can also change community norms around schizophrenia and associated stigma. In this way, peer support can potentially mitigate stigmatized beliefs such as that people with schizophrenia are dangerous or that they are not productive members of society. At the organizational level, embedding peer supporters in mental health services, where patients receive their care, brings an important perspective of lived experience to the care team. On the interpersonal level, peer support addresses the very real phenomenon of social isolation and provides concrete support to those living with schizophrenia. Additionally, peer support interventions can result in improved patient-provider communication and collaboration. For individuals, peer support can have positive effects on treatment adherence, symptoms and functioning, quality of life, patient activation, and recovery-related outcomes. It can also promote appropriate use of routine mental health services and decrease the use of acute care services.

These outcomes of peer support, in turn, influence the availability and potency of the needed inputs for successful peer support services. For example, policy advocacy efforts drive institutional changes, such as policies that require insurance coverage of peer support services and mandate that mental health services be recovery focused. As peer support services impact the organizations and communities in which they operate, community and organizational capacity to implement and sustain these activities grows. Individually and interpersonally, people who have benefited from peer support services and have gained experience in successfully managing their mental health condition are excellent candidates to become peer supporters themselves. In these ways, the outcomes of peer support influence the inputs, creating a positive feedback loop.

3.8 Summary and Implications

Peer support as a concept is richly informed by many theoretical ideas and traditions. These theoretical underpinnings allow for an intuitive understanding of how and why peer support can assist in promoting recovery among those diagnosed with schizophrenia. However, conceptual models specifically outlining how peer support activities are intended to function to promote recovery and better mental health outcomes are lacking in the literature. Theorized mechanisms of change are rarely explicated in research and even less commonly measured. Without a clear idea of how peer supporters provide their services and the ways in which this provision differs from that of professional helpers, building an evidence base for peer support in mental health services has proven to be difficult [53].

Peer supporters are trained to connect with the people they serve by using their shared lived experience in ways that professionals are not trained to do; however, few studies describe or measure these mechanisms [53]. Translating this broad theoretical understanding of peer support to specific and measurable constructs would allow for the empirical investigation of the seemingly intuitive workings of peer support interventions. The lack of such change models is identified as a limitation of many trials of peer support interventions in mental health [54]. Thus, the primary aim of the research presented in this book is to better understand the theoretical constructs that, explicitly or implicitly, underlie peer support programs.

References

1. Cohen S. Social relationships and health. Am Psychol. 2004;59(8):676.
2. Cohen S, Wills TA. Stress, social support, and the buffering hypothesis. Psychol Bull. 1985;98(2):310.
3. Holt-Lunstad J, Smith TB, Layton JB. Social relationships and mortality risk: a meta-analytic review. PLoS Med. 2010;7(7):e1000316.
4. House JS, Landis KR, Umberson D. Social relationships and health. Science. 1988;241(4865):540–5.
5. Strine TW, Chapman DP, Balluz L, Mokdad AH. Health-related quality of life and health behaviors by social and emotional support. Soc Psychiatry Psychiatr Epidemiol. 2008;43(2):151–9.
6. Uchino BN. Social support and physical health: understanding the health consequences of relationships. Yale University Press; 2004.
7. Leigh-Hunt N, Bagguley D, Bash K, Turner V, Turnbull S, Valtorta N, et al. An overview of systematic reviews on the public health consequences of social isolation and loneliness. Public Health. 2017;152:157–71.
8. Holt-Lunstad J, Smith TB, Baker M, Harris T, Stephenson D. Loneliness and social isolation as risk factors for mortality: a meta-analytic review. Perspect Psychol Sci. 2015;10(2):227–37.
9. Gonzalez JS, Penedo FJ, Antoni MH, Durán RE, McPherson-Baker S, Ironson G, et al. Social support, positive states of mind, and HIV treatment adherence in men and women living with HIV/AIDS. Health Psychol. 2004;23(4):413.
10. Catz SL, Kelly JA, Bogart LM, Benotsch EG, McAuliffe TL. Patterns, correlates, and barriers to medication adherence among persons prescribed new treatments for HIV disease. Health Psychol. 2000;19(2):124.

11. Stentzel U, van den Berg N, Schulze LN, Schwaneberg T, Radicke F, Langosch JM, et al. Predictors of medication adherence among patients with severe psychiatric disorders: findings from the baseline assessment of a randomized controlled trial (Tecla). BMC Psychiatry. 2018;18(1):1–8.
12. Fiore M. Treating tobacco use and dependence: 2008 update: clinical practice guideline. Diane Publishing; 2008.
13. van den Brand FA, Nagtzaam P, Nagelhout GE, Winkens B, van Schayck CP. The association of peer smoking behavior and social support with quit success in employees who participated in a smoking cessation intervention at the workplace. Int J Environ Res Public Health. 2019;16(16):2831.
14. Wing RR, Jeffery RW. Benefits of recruiting participants with friends and increasing social support for weight loss and maintenance. J Consult Clin Psychol. 1999;67(1):132.
15. Gorin A, Phelan S, Tate D, Sherwood N, Jeffery R, Wing R. Involving support partners in obesity treatment. J Consult Clin Psychol. 2005;73(2):341.
16. Holt-Lunstad J. Why social relationships are important for physical health: a systems approach to understanding and modifying risk and protection. Annu Rev Psychol. 2018;69:437–58.
17. Heaney CA, Israel BA. Social networks and social support. In: Health behavior and health education: theory, research, and practice, vol. 4; 2008. p. 189–210.
18. Berkman LF, Glass T. Social integration, social networks, social support, and health. Soci Epidemiol. 2000;1:137–73.
19. House JS. Work stress and social support. 1981.
20. Kowitt SD, Urlaub D, Guzman-Corrales L, Mayer M, Ballesteros J, Graffy J, et al. Emotional support for diabetes management: an international cross-cultural study. Diabetes Educ. 2015;41(3):291–300.
21. Repper J, Aldridge B, Gilfoyle S, Gillard S, Perkins R, Rennison J. Peer support workers: theory and practice. Citeseer; 2013.
22. Kowitt S, Yu S, Owens AK, Carey LA, Fisher EB. Social support needs among patients with advanced breast cancer: sensitivity trumps substance. J Commu Support Oncol. 2016;14(12):509–14.
23. Fisher E, Bickle C, Harber K, Hughes C, Jeffe D, Kahl L, et al. Benefits of directive and nondirective support are moderated by severity of circumstances. San Francisco: Annual Meeting of Society of Behavioral Medicine; 1997.
24. Gabriele JM, Carpenter BD, Tate DF, Fisher EB. Directive and nondirective e-coach support for weight loss in overweight adults. Ann Behav Med. 2010;41(2):252–63.
25. Evans M, Fisher EB. Social isolation and mental health: the role of nondirective and directive social support. Community Ment Health J. 2021;58:20. https://doi.org/10.1007/s10597-021-00787-9.
26. Fisher EB, Bhushan NL, Coufal MM, Kowitt SD, Parada H, Sokol RL, et al. Peer support in prevention, chronic disease management, and Well-being. In: Principles and concepts of behavioral medicine. Springer; 2018. p. 643–77.
27. Oborn E, Barrett M, Gibson S, Gillard S. Knowledge and expertise in care practices: the role of the peer worker in mental health teams. Sociol Health Illn. 2019;41:1305.
28. Bandura A. Social learning theory. Englewood Cliffs: Prentice Hall; 1977.
29. McAlister AL, Perry CL, Parcel GS, Glanz K, Rimer BK, Viswanath K. Health behavior and health education: theory, research, and practice. In: How individuals, environments, and health behaviors interact: social cognitive theory; 2008.
30. Schunck D. Peer models and children's behavior change. Rev Educ Res. 1987;57:149–74.
31. Festinger L. A theory of social comparison processes. Hum Relat. 1954;7(2):117–40.
32. Kotera Y, Llewellyn-Beardsley J, Charles A, Slade M. Common humanity as an under-acknowledged mechanism for mental health peer support. Int J Ment Heal Addict. 2022:1–7. https://doi.org/10.1007/s11469-022-00916-9.
33. Goffman E. Asylums: essays on the social situation of mental patrients and other innates. Dubledzay; 1961.

34. Rosenhan DL. On being sane in insane places. Science. 1973;179(4070):250–8.
35. Smith TE, Easter A, Pollock M, Pope LG, Wisdom JP. Disengagement from care: perspectives of individuals with serious mental illness and of service providers. Psychiatr Serv. 2013;64(8):770–5.
36. Link BG, Phelan JC. Labeling and stigma. In: Handbook of the sociology of mental health. Springer; 2013. p. 525–41.
37. Corrigan PW, Druss BG, Perlick DA. The impact of mental illness stigma on seeking and participating in mental health care. Psychol Sci Public Interest. 2014;15(2):37–70.
38. Schulze B. Stigma and mental health professionals: a review of the evidence on an intricate relationship. Int Rev Psychiatry. 2007;19(2):137–55.
39. Fisher EB, Earp JA, Maman S, Zolotor A. Cross-cultural and international adaptation of peer support for diabetes management. Fam Pract. 2009;27(suppl_1):i6–i16.
40. Fisher EB, Boothroyd RI, Coufal MM, Baumann LC, Mbanya JC, Rotheram-Borus MJ, et al. Peer support for self-management of diabetes improved outcomes in international settings. Health Aff. 2012;31(1):130–9.
41. Evans M, Daaleman TP, Fisher EB. Peer support for chronic medical conditions. In: Avery J, editor. Peer support in medicine: a quick guide. New York: Springer; 2021. p. 49–70.
42. Fisher EB, Ballesteros J, Bhushan N, Coufal MM, Kowitt SD, McDonough AM, et al. Key features of peer support in chronic disease prevention and management. Health Aff. 2015;34(9):1523–30.
43. Fisher EB, Tang PY, Evans M, Bhushan N, Graham MA, Valovcin DD, et al. The fundamental value of presence in peer and mutual support: observations from telephone support for high risk groups. Global J Commu Psychol Pract. 2020;11(3):1–20.
44. Plett H. The art of holding space: a practice of love, liberation, and leadership. Page Two Books, Incorporated; 2020.
45. Kahlon MK, Aksan N, Aubrey R, Clark N, Cowley-Morillo M, Jacobs EA, et al. Effect of layperson-delivered, empathy-focused program of telephone calls on loneliness, depression, and anxiety among adults during the COVID-19 pandemic: a randomized clinical trial. JAMA Psychiatry. 2021;78(6):616–22.
46. Thorpe CT, Fahey LE, Johnson H, Deshpande M, Thorpe JM, Fisher EB. Facilitating healthy coping in patients with diabetes: a systematic review. Diabetes Educ. 2013;39(1):33–52.
47. Peers for Progress. Global evidence for peer support: humanizing health care. Report from an International Conference hosted by Peers for Progress and the National Council of La Raza. American Academy of Family Physicians Foundation. Leawood, 2014.
48. Pickett SA, Diehl SM, Steigman PJ, Prater JD, Fox A, Shipley P, et al. Consumer empowerment and self-advocacy outcomes in a randomized study of peer-led education. Community Ment Health J. 2012;48(4):420–30.
49. del Vecchio P. Peer service providers as colleagues. In: Handbook of community psychiatry. Springer; 2012. p. 117–23.
50. Lorig K, Ritter PL, Plant K. A disease-specific self-help program compared with a generalized chronic disease self-help program for arthritis patients. Arthritis Rheum. 2005;53(6):950–7.
51. Earp JA, Eng E, O'Malley MS, Altpeter M, Rauscher G, Mayne L, et al. Increasing use of mammography among older, rural African American women: results from a community trial. Am J Public Health. 2002;92(4):646–54.
52. Sallis JF, Owen N, Fisher E. Ecological models of health behavior. Health Behav Theory Res Pract. 2015;5:43–64.
53. Bellamy C, Schmutte T, Davidson L. An update on the growing evidence base for peer support. Ment Health Soc Incl. 2017;21(3):161–7.
54. Pitt V, Lowe D, Hill S, Prictor M, Hetrick SE, Ryan R, et al. Consumer-providers of care for adult clients of statutory mental health services. Cochrane Database Syst Rev. 2013;2013:CD004807.

Chapter 4
Origins of Peer Support and the Modern Recovery Movement in the United States

> The concept of recovery is rooted in the simple yet profound realization that people who have been diagnosed with a mental illness are human beings. (Patricia Deegan 1995)

Psychiatry and other mental health professions contend with a dark past, in which people experiencing mental illness were housed in institutions that either offered no treatment, ineffective treatment, or well-intentioned treatment that nevertheless caused harm [1]. People living with mental illnesses were thought to be incurable, with hopeless futures that most likely involved destitution, institutionalization, incarceration, and early death [1]. Certainly, little hope is found in Emil Kraeplin's conceptualization of "dementia praecox," a disorder marked by progressive deterioration into a "permanent state of psychological weakness" [2]. Throughout history, people with mental illnesses have organized to push back against these views, and while they have achieved many gains, the work continues. This chapter presents an abbreviated history of the origins of peer support and the modern recovery movement in the United States.

4.1 Moral Treatment

First, often cited as the earliest example of peer support is the work of Phillippe Pinel and Jean-Baptiste Pussin in eighteenth-century France. Pussin, a former patient of the hospital, and Pinel, the hospital's chief physician, banned the use of chains on wards for mentally ill patients and replaced them with treatment practices thought to be more humane [3]. The wards were staffed by former patients who were valued for making services more civilized, caring, and kind [3]. This began what is known as the moral treatment era [3], with the term "moral" meaning "mental" or "psychological" [4, 5]. During this era, it was first posited that psychological, behavioral, social, and environmental factors could be therapeutically manipulated to alleviate mental suffering [4, 5]. Previously, treatments were primarily physical, such as bloodletting and immobilization [4]. One critic of this optimistic

M. Evans, *Peer Support Services Reaching People with Schizophrenia*,
https://doi.org/10.1007/978-3-031-29042-8_4

interpretation of Pinel, Michel Foucault, noted that while mental patients were no longer chained to the walls, they were nonetheless still confined [6]. Nevertheless, the moral treatment era is considered an important period in the history of mental health care and treatment.

4.2 Institutionalization and Associated Human Rights Abuses

Several influential thought leaders in the nineteenth and early twentieth centuries brought attention to the injustices and human rights abuses which often occurred in mental institutions. In England in 1845, former asylum patients and their supporters formed the Alleged Lunatic's Friend Society and campaigned against wrongful confinement and cruel treatment [7]. In the period following the American Civil War in the United States, Elizabeth Packard formed the Anti-Insane Asylum Society after being forcibly detained at an asylum on the recommendation of her husband [7]. Around the same time, Elizabeth Stone, who was also committed to an asylum by her husband, led organizing efforts to influence public opinion and stop unjust incarceration of the mentally ill [7]. In 1907, Clifford Beers wrote an influential book, *A Mind That Found Itself,* based on his experiences of mental illness and institutionalization. He then founded the National Committee for Mental Hygiene, now known as Mental Health America [7, 8]. Although initially outspoken about abuse of mental patients and critical of psychiatrists for their tolerance of this mistreatment, Beers eventually concluded that his reform movement would be more successful if it included leading psychiatrists [9, 10]. After their inclusion, the group quickly became dominated by professionals [10, 11].

4.3 Deinstitutionalization

Deinstitutionalization, the radical restructuring of mental health care that took place between 1950 and 1970 in the United States, laid the groundwork for the modern recovery movement. Importantly, the development of psychotropic drugs called into question the need for and utility of long-term institutionalization [12]. Furthering the process, the Community Mental Health Act, which promised funding for community facilities to serve people with mental disabilities, was signed into law by President John F. Kennedy in 1963 [12]. It is thought that Kennedy was invested in this cause due to his personal experience with his sister, who had been lobotomized at 23 upon her father's request [12]. Shortly after the passage of this Act, however, President Kennedy was assassinated and the funds to increase community alternatives to psychiatric hospitalization never materialized to the extent they were promised. Thus, many people with mental illnesses were freed from institutions, but the infrastructure to provide them care in the community was underdeveloped. This dearth of community care options led to many people with mental illnesses becoming unhoused or incarcerated. At the same time, however, people who were formerly institutionalized began to meet and organize.

4.4 Organized Civil Rights and the Growth of the Recovery Movement

Heavily influenced by the organized efforts of other civil rights movements of the time including Black civil rights, women's rights, gay rights, and disability rights, the movement truly took off in the early 1970s [7, 9]. On the heels of deinstitutionalization, former patients began to organize and assert a new entitlement to speak on their own behalf [11]. The inhumane conditions and treatment practices many experienced at mental institutions led to ex-patients organizing to liberate themselves and others from this system. Their first goal was not to reform the mental health system but rather to shut it down [11]. The name of the first consumer-run rights group for mental patients, the Oregon Insane Liberation Front, highlights this objective [11]. Groups such as these developed in many different cities across the United States and engaged in protests and demonstrations aimed at bringing attention to and, ultimately, terminating coercive treatment practices that led to human rights abuses. Early protestors began to communicate with each other by means of a national newsletter, *Madness Network News*, and holding annual conferences, and, as a result, a national movement was born [10, 11].

This movement pushed for alternatives to traditional mental health care. In 1978, Judi Chamberlin wrote the book *On Our Own: Patient-Controlled Alternatives to the Mental Health System*, in which she argued that people with mental illnesses should direct their own care and pushed back on traditional notions of compliance [13]. From her perspective, recovery, or being able to live fully and independently, was the goal of mental health treatment, not compliance with medications or other treatments [13]. Consumer choice was paramount and chosen services often included other people with lived experience of mental illness [13]. Reflecting the organized civil rights movements that influenced her thinking, Chamberlin underscored the importance of consciousness raising in creating real alternatives to mental health treatment [13]. She viewed partnership models in which patients and providers work together to provide services as alternatives in name only [13]. In her view, true alternatives are provided only by supportive models, in which membership is open to all people who want to use the service for mutual support and professionals are excluded except in external roles, and separatist models, in which all support and services are provided by ex-patients [13].

4.5 Organizing of Families of People with Mental Illnesses

In 1979, at the same time as the consumer/survivor/ex-patient movement was gaining momentum, another advocacy group the National Alliance for the Mentally Ill (NAMI) was formed [7, 11]. Founded by family members of people with mental illness, NAMI grew quickly and was successful in securing funds to advance research on the biological origins of mental illness [10]. In pursuit of their aim to reduce stigma and change the perception of mental illness as caused by poor parenting, NAMI forged close ties with the American Psychiatric Association, National Institute of Mental Health, and the pharmaceutical industry [14]. Together, these organizations worked to advance the conceptualization of mental illness as biologically based brain disease [14]. There was tension between the consumer/survivor/ex-patient movement and the organization of families, some of which remains today [10]. Some consumers questioned the legitimacy of families' perspectives on treatment, which tended to be more paternalistic than preferences of consumers themselves [10]. Traditional mental health associations struggled to adapt to activism from both families and patients [10].

4.6 Ideological Differences and Debates

The growth of the movement was not without challenges and disagreements among different factions. Several ideological differences are important to consider as they continue to influence perspectives on mental health in the present day. First, some thought the movement should be outer focused, a social movement, while others preferred an inner focused, individual therapy approach. Other important issues arose around the nature of mental illness and the utility of mental health treatment. Among these critical issues was the concept of separatism. Different individuals and groups disagreed whether to include or exclude mental health professionals, family members, and others without experience of mental illness [10]. The separatist approach viewed psychiatry as antithetical to its goals and was opposed to inclusion of mental health professionals within its ranks. On the other hand, more moderate factions wanted to build a broad coalition and viewed the inclusion of mental health professionals more pragmatically. Furthermore, the extent to which members and factions of the movement agreed with or saw the utility in the medical model of mental illness differed. Some viewed treatment as necessary and useful, if in need of serious reform, while others aimed to abolish the institution of psychiatry in its entirety.

Finally, there were rhetorical disagreements [9]. Three important terms warrant distinction: consumer, survivor, and ex-patient. The term "consumer" describes those who receive services and generally accept the medical model of mental illness; the term "survivor" refers to individuals who recount terrible experiences with mental health care and want little to do with it going forward; and the term "ex-patient" designates individuals who are simply glad they got away [10, 15].

Mental health consumer is the term most often used in the United States currently; however, many of those who were involved in the early recovery movement preferred the term psychiatric survivor, or even ex-psychiatric inmate, reflecting a more militant stance [9, 10].

These rhetorical debates continued as the movement grew and became more mainstream, less radical, and more cooperative with psychiatry [9, 10]. The "ex-inmate/ex-patient" movement transformed from one that was generally anti-medical model and emancipatory to the "consumer/survivor" movement, a more organized, although also more politically divergent group whose members were willing to work with the mental health system and government agencies [10]. Consumerism, with its focus on choice in services, and recovery rhetoric are the dominant ideologies of the movement in recent years [10, 16]. However, the term consumer has been criticized as implying that people with mental illnesses are a burden on society and centers their identity on the receipt of mental health services [17]. The term person with a psychiatric disability has been suggested as a more accurate and appropriate expression [5, 17].

4.7 Recovery in the Mainstream

Decades of organizing resulted in important reforms to the mental health system. In 2003, the President's New Freedom Commission on Mental Health was released, stating that mental health care should be "recovery oriented," meaning that services should be collaborative and respectful and should emphasize attaining a satisfying life even in the presence of mental illness symptoms [18]. This shift to recovery-oriented care was influenced by the recognition that, while full clinical recovery was possible, a more personal sense of recovery was required for others and that mental health care was primarily focused on acute care to alleviate signs and symptoms of disorder and paid considerably less attention to promoting individual and community functioning [19]. Recovery-oriented care involves institutional change, with more emphasis on choice, person-centered care, and shared decision-making, especially in respect to medication [20]. Definitions of recovery have evolved throughout the years and have been criticized as being co-opted by neoliberalism and capitalism [19]. The extent to which recovery transformation has been achieved throughout the mental health care system in the United States has not been empirically evaluated and likely varies considerably across locations and settings.

4.8 Growth of Formal Peer Support Services

Following the President's New Freedom Commission on Mental Health report, the Department of Veterans Affairs started funding positions for veterans with lived experience of mental health issues to provide support services to other veterans with SMI in 2005 [21]. Certified peer specialists first became Medicaid reimbursable in

Georgia in 2007 and have since increased exponentially in the provision of mental health care, with at least 35 states' Medicaid programs now covering them as a reimbursable service [22]. This development was particularly important, as Medicaid is the single largest payer for mental health services in the United States (Centers for Medicare and Medicaid Services, 2019). Forty-five states have peer support specialist certification programs [23], and in 2022, President Biden included building a national certification program for peer specialists as part of his strategy to address the national mental health crisis in the United States [24]. These developments suggest that that formal peer support services will continue to proliferate in the coming years.

4.9 Summary

Peer support and the modern recovery movement have historical roots dating back to the eighteenth century. In the United States, deinstitutionalization and other organized civil rights movements influenced the growth of the modern recovery movement, which has achieved many gains in making mental health care more humane. One important practice to emerge from this movement was the inclusion of formal peer support services in mental health care. These services, and especially their use among people with schizophrenia or other psychoses, are the basis of the research described in the remaining chapters.

References

1. Davidson L, White W. The concept of recovery as an organizing principle for integrating mental health and addiction services. J Behav Health Serv Res. 2007;34(2):109–20.
2. Read J, Mosher LR, Bentall RP. Models of madness: psychological, social and biological approaches to schizophrenia. Psychology Press. Hove, East Sussex, UK. 2004.
3. Davidson L, Bellamy C, Guy K, Miller R. Peer support among persons with severe mental illnesses: a review of evidence and experience. World Psychiatry. 2012;11(2):123–8.
4. Charland L. Moral treatment. In: The encyclopedia of clinical psychology. Wiley-Blackwell; 2015. https://doi.org/10.1002/9781118625392wbecp094.
5. Davidson L, Rakfeldt J, Strauss J. The roots of the recovery movement in psychiatry: lessons learned. Wiley. Chichester, West Sussex, UK. 2011.
6. Foucault M. Madness and civilization. Antipsychiatry Movement 1964:86.
7. Frese FJ, Davis WW. The consumer–survivor movement, recovery, and consumer professionals. Prof Psychol Res Pract. 1997;28(3):243.
8. Beers CW. A mind that found itself. 1907.
9. Chamberlin J. The ex-patients' movement: where we've been and where we're going. J Mind Behavior. 1990;11:323–36.
10. McLean AH. From ex-patient alternatives to consumer options: consequences of consumerism for psychiatric consumers and the ex-patient movement. Int J Health Serv. 2000;30(4):821–47.
11. Tomes N. The patient as a policy factor: a historical case study of the consumer/survivor movement in mental health. Health Aff. 2006;25(3):720–9.

12. Erickson B. Deinstitutionalization through optimism: the community mental health act of 1963. Am J Psychiatry Resid J. 2021;16:6.
13. Chamberlin J. On our own: patient-controlled alternatives to the mental health system. McGraw-Hill; 1978.
14. Deacon BJ. The biomedical model of mental disorder: a critical analysis of its validity, utility, and effects on psychotherapy research. Clin Psychol Rev. 2013;33(7):846–61.
15. Rosenthal H. Transformative impact and initiatives of the mental health consumer/survivor movement. In: Service delivery for vulnerable populations: new directions in behavioral health. New York: Springer; 2010. p. 415–29.
16. Braslow JT. The manufacture of recovery. Annu Rev Clin Psychol. 2013;9:781–809.
17. Hensley MA. Why I am not a "mental health consumer". Psychiatr Rehabil J. 2006;30(1):67.
18. President's New Freedom Commission on Mental Health. Achieving the promise: transforming mental health care in America. 2003.
19. Davidson L, Rowe M, DiLeo P, Bellamy C, Delphin-Rittmon M. Recovery-oriented systems of care: a perspective on the past, present, and future. Alcohol Res. 2021;41(1):9.
20. Slade M, Amering M, Farkas M, Hamilton B, O'Hagan M, Panther G, et al. Uses and abuses of recovery: implementing recovery-oriented practices in mental health systems. World Psychiatry. 2014;13(1):12–20.
21. Chinman M, Lucksted A, Gresen R, Davis M, Losonczy M, Sussner B, et al. Early experiences of employing consumer-providers in the VA. Psychiatr Serv. 2008;59(11):1315–21.
22. Copeland Center for Wellness and Recovery I: How are peer support services paid for by the state? What specific Medicaid waivers are used, if any? In: Peer specialist database. https://copelandcenter.com/peer-specialists (2022). Accessed 23 Aug 2022.
23. Copeland Center for Wellness and Recovery I: Is there a state-wide certification test? In: Peer specialist database. https://copelandcenter.com/peer-specialists (2022). Accessed 23 Aug 2022.
24. Canady VA. President Biden's national strategy to support MH workforce, address crisis. Ment Heal Wkly. 2022;32(10):1–3. https://doi.org/10.1002/mhw.33138.
25. Deegan P. Recovery as a journey of the heart. Psychiatric rehabilitation journal. 1995;19(3):91.

Chapter 5
Peer Support and Mental Health: A Review of the Evidence

As peer support services continue to proliferate in practice, the evidence base has not kept pace and has been described as "frustratingly messy" [1, 2]. Findings of effectiveness are largely mixed, likely due at least in part to the continued confusion and lack of clarity about the definition of peer support services [3]. Reviewers frequently recommend more rigorous research and better reporting of interventions and outcomes [3]. Methodological limitations as well as significant variability in programs and participants contribute to the unclear nature of the evidence [3]. While adaptability and variety in peer support services are undoubtedly assets that assist in the success of these programs in varied settings, significant heterogeneity of interventions makes evidence synthesis difficult [4, 5].

The literature reports a wide variability of peer support activities provided [6] and no generally agreed upon outcomes to measure [7]. Peer support is conceptualized and delivered in a wide range of formats [8], including protocolized interventions delivered at least in part by a peer supporter [9, 10], traditional mental health services with at least one peer supporter on the service team [11–13], Internet psychoeducation programs [14, 15] and befriending programs [16]. The outcomes measured vary widely and include recovery, hopefulness, empowerment, quality of life, patient activation, mental illness symptoms, hospitalizations, arrests, emergency room visits, engagement with care, satisfaction with care, and global functioning [5]. These considerations, along with the variability in the term mental health itself, have made synthesizing the evidence a challenge.

5.1 Review of Systematic Reviews and Meta-Analyses

Several systematic reviews and meta-analyses warrant attention. First, Pitt and colleagues (2013) conducted a meta-analysis of 11 randomized controlled trials (RCT) from 1979 to 2012 involving *consumer providers* comparing consumer staff to

M. Evans, *Peer Support Services Reaching People with Schizophrenia*, https://doi.org/10.1007/978-3-031-29042-8_5

professional staff in the same roles or comparing mental health services with or without consumer-providers as an adjunct to the service. Their results show that services provided by consumer providers achieved psychosocial, mental health, and service use outcomes that are comparable with professional staff [17]. The authors concluded that there was low-quality evidence to suggest that consumer-provided services in mental health teams resulted in a small reduction in clients' use of crisis or emergency services [17].

Another review by Lloyd-Evans and colleagues (2014) consisted of a meta-analysis of 18 RCTs from 1982 to 2013 which included *mutual support groups* ($n = 4$), *peer support services* ($n = 11$), or *peer mental health providers* ($n = 3$). The authors identified some serious risk of bias in all but two of the studies examined and, from the available evidence, concluded that there is little evidence that peer support improves service users' hospitalization, overall symptoms, or satisfaction outcomes [5]. Some evidence did suggest that peer support is associated with benefit on measures more directly related to a recovery process such as hope and empowerment [5].

Fuhr and colleagues (2014) conducted a meta-analysis of 14 RCTs for SMI ($n = 10$) and depression ($n = 4$) comparing *peer services* to treatment as usual (superiority trials) or to services provided by health professionals (equivalence trials). Results from two of the equivalence trials suggest that peers are as effective as professional staff regarding symptom and quality of life improvements [18]. Additionally, results from three high-quality superiority trials showed small positive effects that favored peer-delivered interventions on quality of life and hope [18].

Chinman and colleagues conducted a systematic review of 20 studies from 1995 to 2012, which included 11 RCTs and 9 quasi-experimental or correlational studies evaluating three types of interventions: *peers added to traditional services, peers in existing clinical roles,* and *peers delivering structured curricula.* Overall, the level of evidence for each type of peer support service was moderate and effectiveness varied by type of intervention [19]. Compared with professional staff, peers added to traditional services or providing curricula were associated with reduced inpatient use and an improvement in a range of recovery outcomes; however, evidence of peers in existing roles was mixed [19].

Fisher and colleagues, in a review of peer support interventions for a broad range of health behaviors and outcomes, found that six of eight studies that focused on mental health problems, including postpartum depression, had outcomes that favored peer support. Five of these trials showed significant between-group differences favoring peer support, and one showed significant within-group changes [20].

Most recently, White and colleagues conducted a systematic review and meta-analysis of one-to-one peer support for adults using mental health services. They reviewed 23 papers describing 19 unique peer support interventions and reported a modest, positive effect on empowerment and self-reported recovery [4]. Results of the meta-analysis suggested no improvement in clinical outcomes and suggest that the benefits of peer support are largely psychosocial [4]. While this review took a more focused approach, the authors still reported significant heterogeneity in intervention approaches and outcomes [4].

5.2 The Distinctive Contributions of Peer Support

In conventional mental health roles, such as case management, most studies find that peer staff function as well as non-peer staff, with comparable outcomes [21, 22]. Additionally, peer-delivered services have been shown to be superior in engaging "difficult to reach" clients [22]. Qualitative findings show that people with mental illnesses view their relationships with peer supporters as nonhierarchical and nonclinical, in contrast to their relationships with conventional mental health providers [23, 24]. Overall, however, less is known about the unique contributions of peer-delivered services and how peers may perform their roles differently from non-peer staff.

Thus far, the literature has suggested that peer-delivered services may be unique in their ability to instill hope through positive self-disclosure and use role modeling and experiential knowledge to address self-care behaviors and negotiate day-to-day life with a mental illness [25]. Social comparison theory underscores the importance of comparing others with our own sense of self and partly explains how peer interventions can help recipients by providing an example of a person successfully recovering [26]. Additionally, social learning theory purports that if an individual sees someone like them succeed, this role modeling experience can increase their own self-efficacy and self-esteem [27, 28]. This observational learning is a key underpinning of peer support interventions. Peer supporters acting as positive role models may also reduce mental illness stigma in a variety of ways, from combatting self-stigma in consumers to challenging stigma among clinicians.

The lived experience of the peer supporter has the potential to inform the way services are delivered to address concerns such as with housing, transportation, and finances that may be related to, yet separate from, psychological issues like symptoms and functioning. Tangible support such as this should not be discounted in its ability to aid recovery by reducing stress and worry and providing a foundation for the more therapeutic aspects of the peer support relationship [24]. Peer supporters may help their clients advocate for themselves in their interactions with mental health treatment providers [24]. Additionally, the peer provider may be well situated to have a relationship with their clients characterized by trust, acceptance, understanding, and empathy, enhancing the other aspects of the peer support relationship [25].

5.3 Current Evidence Regarding Peer Support in the Treatment of Schizophrenia

The participation of consumers in the planning, delivery, and evaluation of services is increasingly recognized as essential to recovery-oriented services for persons with schizophrenia and related psychoses [29]. While peer-based services have not yet met the Schizophrenia Patient Outcomes Research Team (PORT) standard for a psychosocial treatment recommendation for people with schizophrenia, they do show evidence of being a promising intervention for recovery [29]. Unfortunately, the research literature in this area to date is small and limited by weak experimental designs [29]. However, both peer support and schizophrenia are perhaps best viewed as categories and not evaluated as single entities. For example, when considering improvement in schizophrenia, one could consider improvement in symptoms, positive or negative, improvement in social functioning, improvement in mood, as well as improvement in life circumstances such as housing status and employment. Likewise, peer support is too broad and varied an approach to be sufficiently evaluated as a single thing.

While peer support has been widely studied in chronic disease and mental health broadly, far less research has focused on peer support specifically for people diagnosed with schizophrenia or those with experience of psychosis. In a recent systematic review examining the effectiveness of peer support interventions on hospital admission, relapse, global state, quality of life, death, and cost to society for people with schizophrenia, there were only 13 trials identified for inclusion, and only two of the specified outcomes were measured [30]. The available evidence was deemed to be of low quality, and the authors concluded that there is insufficient high-quality evidence available to either support or refute the effectiveness of peer support for people with schizophrenia [30]. Notable exceptions to this general lack of evidence in this area are reviewed below.

Two instances of peer support groups for people with schizophrenia or other psychoses have been empirically evaluated. First, peer-led mutual support groups for people with schizophrenia and their families in China demonstrated favorable outcomes, with patients randomized to the support group condition reporting consistently greater improvements over 3 years in overall functioning and reductions in duration and number of hospitalizations [31–34]. It is important to note that the peers in these studies were family members of people with schizophrenia and not those with the disorder themselves. Minimally guided mutual support groups for adults with psychotic disorders in the Netherlands demonstrated positive effects on contact with peers outside of sessions and esteem support [35, 36]. These groups were led by a nurse but based on a minimal guidance structure, with the nurse's main role being to facilitate interaction between group members. Subgroup analyses of completers showed that high attenders had significant improvements in social support, self-efficacy, and quality of life compared to low attenders, indicating a dose-response relationship [36].

There were also two empirical evaluations of individual peer support focused primarily on people with schizophrenia and other psychotic disorders. In a quasi-experimental study of telephone-based peer support for people diagnosed with schizophrenia in Australia, Boardman and colleagues (2014) reported that participants improved in medication adherence and total symptoms over a period of 14 weeks. They also observed a reduction in negative symptoms between baseline and 8 weeks [37]. In a pilot study conducted in Germany, peer counseling for consumers in a specialized open ward for inpatients with schizophrenia and schizoaffective disorders was widely accepted, with 96% of participants reporting that they would definitely advise other patients on the ward to take part in the consultation [38]. Participants reported liking the following aspects of the counseling: "understanding of or trust in the peer-counselor" (40%), "advice by a peer" (18%), "openness of the counselor" (17%), "information on schizophrenia and medication" (17%), and "active listening of the peer-counselor" (12%) [38].

As a precursor to this research, I conducted a systematic scoping review of the published literature on peer-delivered services and peer support reaching people with schizophrenia [8]. The review included 22 studies describing 20 unique interventions. Half were not restricted to people with schizophrenia and instead were provided to mixed-diagnosis groups, suggesting that tailoring programs for diagnosis-specific needs may be warranted [8]. Additionally, three of four studies that measured negative symptoms reported significant changes favoring peer services [8]. Surprisingly, given the priority placed on ongoing adherence and community placement among this population, only half of programs provided ongoing support, operationalized liberally as follows: (1) support conveniently and directly available on an ongoing basis throughout the duration of the observation period with a minimum of 3 months or (2) programs lasting at least 12 months [8]. Several omissions in the content of peer programs included the absence of vocational, educational, and housing outcomes which are acknowledged as vitally important to recovery [8]. Results illustrate that peer-delivered services and peer support are diverse categories and, thus, future research should evaluate the specific strategies and activities employed by peers to allow for a greater understanding of what works for whom in this area [8].

5.4 Potential for Peer Support to Promote Recovery Among People with Schizophrenia

Although current research is inconclusive, there are several hypothesized ways peer support may be effective at advancing recovery among people with schizophrenia. Promoting engagement in treatment, advocating for consumer needs and preferences, and linking people with needed services are potential strategies that complement comprehensive mental health care [39]. Additionally, peer support may increase social skills and connections, decrease social isolation, combat stigma, and help address concrete issues such as housing and employment. The research presented here reviews the vast and diverse literature on the subject to elucidate the peer support strategies, document benefits of these strategies, and suggest potential mechanisms linking strategy to benefit.

5.5 Research Gaps and Implications

RCTs, systematic reviews, and meta-analyses may not be the best tools to understand the nuances of how and why peer support programs impact mental health recovery. Heavily grounded in the biomedical paradigm, RCTs treat complex social interventions as akin to straightforward medical treatments and aim to control for all context-specific variation, which, in the case of social programs, is always present and heavily impacts the successes or failures demonstrated by each individual program [40]. Thus, a meta-analysis pooling results from RCTs is heavily focused on the question of "does it work?" and does not consider "how it works, for whom, and in what circumstances?" [40]. Understanding of these nuances is critical to the success of complex social interventions such as peer support and, thus, RCTs and meta-analyses may not be best to understand complex interventions [40]. Thus, the approach taken here— a realist review of the literature— utilizes evidence from a variety of data sources to provide insight into the complex nature of peer support programs and their theoretical underpinnings [41]. It intends to provide explanations of how programs work as opposed to a judgment of whether peer support as a single entity works or does not work [40].

Furthermore, continued research is needed to better understand the work activities of peer support specialists in different contexts so that we can assess the quality of these services [43]. This research pays close attention to the specific peer support strategies and activities comprising each peer support intervention, rather than equating all possible activities peers might engage in as "peer support." To provide a detailed and more complete picture of the available evidence describing and evaluating the use of peer support services among people with schizophrenia and related disorders, this research pays close attention to nuance and includes a variety of evidence sources and intervention approaches.

Research on peer support interventions could benefit from theoretical or conceptual models of how the peer support activities delivered are intended to affect the measured outcomes. The background literature search discovered only one such model. Gillard, Gibson, Holley, and Lucock used a grounded theory qualitative approach to develop a change model of peer provided interventions in mental health services [44]. These authors suggest that the first step to effective peer support interventions lies in building trusting relationships based on shared lived experience [44]. Through this, peer supporters can act as role models and bridges between consumers and providers [44]. Shared lived experiences and bridging between consumers and providers are likely to impact these potential mediating factors: hope in the future, empowerment, social functioning, self-care, engagement with services, and strength of social networks [44]. Through these mechanisms of action, peer support services are thought to be able to impact downstream outcomes such as increased recovery, well-being, and service use [44]. Future research should focus on measuring these potential mediators and outcomes of interest to help build an evidence base of how peer support works in addressing mental illness.

5.6 Summary

To summarize, although there is considerable research investigating the effectiveness of peer support for people with mental illnesses, the evidence is mixed and clear recommendations for best practices are elusive. Additionally, the research that has been done often focuses on peer support for mental illness in general and far less on specific diagnostic categories, which are associated with varied challenges and may benefit from varied approaches. Conceptual models and theoretical understanding of how peer support operates to promote recovery and better mental health outcomes are lacking in the literature which further make it difficult to identify the key components, or "active ingredients," of peer support programs.

Nonetheless, peer support programs are proliferating in practice and, thus, research investigating the complex nature of these programs is warranted. Gaining a nuanced understanding of the different peer support activities provided and their benefits will assist program designers, implementers, and key decision-makers to develop services that meet the needs of specific populations. Additionally, there is a need for a better understanding of the mechanisms by which peer support activities are intended to work to lead to improved outcomes for people with schizophrenia. More complete understanding of the complexities of peer support programs will help the field to better implement such supports and to design programs with the potential for maximum impact. The following research addresses these gaps by considering the complexities of peer support and synthesizing knowledge from the published and grey literature with insights from experts in the field.

References

1. Gillard S. Peer support in mental health services: where is the research taking us, and do we want to go there? Taylor & Francis; 2019. p. 341–4.
2. Davidson L. Peer support: coming of age of and/or miles to go before we sleep? An introduction. J Behav Health Serv Res. 2015;42(1):96–9.
3. Bellamy C, Schmutte T, Davidson L. An update on the growing evidence base for peer support. Ment Health Soc Incl. 2017;21(3):161–7.
4. White S, Foster R, Marks J, Morshead R, Goldsmith L, Barlow S, et al. The effectiveness of one-to-one peer support in mental health services: a systematic review and meta-analysis. BMC Psychiatry. 2020;20(1):1–20.
5. Lloyd-Evans B, Mayo-Wilson E, Harrison B, Istead H, Brown E, Pilling S, et al. A systematic review and meta-analysis of randomised controlled trials of peer support for people with severe mental illness. BMC Psychiatry. 2014;14(1):39.
6. Salzer MS, Schwenk E, Brusilovskiy E. Certified peer specialist roles and activities: results from a national survey. Psychiatr Serv. 2010;61(5):520–3.
7. Daniels AS, Bergeson S, Fricks L, Ashenden P, Powell I. Pillars of peer support: advancing the role of peer support specialists in promoting recovery. J Ment Health Train Educ Pract. 2012;7(2):60–9.

8. Evans M, Barker H, Peddireddy S, Zhang A, Luu S, Qian Y, et al. Peer-delivered services and peer support reaching people with schizophrenia: a scoping review. Int J Ment Health. 2021:1–23. https://doi.org/10.1080/00207411.2021.1975441.
9. Barbic S, Krupa T, Armstrong I. A randomized controlled trial of the effectiveness of a modified recovery workbook program: preliminary findings. Psychiatr Serv. 2009;60(4):491–7.
10. Cook JA, Copeland ME, Jonikas JA, Hamilton MM, Razzano LA, Grey DD, et al. Results of a randomized controlled trial of mental illness self-management using Wellness Recovery Action Planning. Schizophr Bull. 2011;38(4):881–91.
11. Chinman M, Oberman RS, Hanusa BH, Cohen AN, Salyers MP, Twamley EW, et al. A cluster randomized trial of adding peer specialists to intensive case management teams in the Veterans Health Administration. J Behav Health Serv Res. 2013;42(1):109–21.
12. Clarke GN, Herinckx HA, Kinney RF, Paulson RI, Cutler DL, Lewis K, et al. Psychiatric hospitalizations, arrests, emergency room visits, and homelessness of clients with serious and persistent mental illness: findings from a randomized trial of two ACT programs vs. usual care. Ment Health Serv Res. 2000;2(3):155–64.
13. Craig T, Doherty I, Jamieson-Craig R, Boocock A, Attafua G. The consumer-employee as a member of a Mental Health Assertive Outreach Team. I. Clinical and social outcomes. J Ment Health. 2004;13(1):59–69.
14. Kaplan K, Salzer MS, Solomon P, Brusilovskiy E, Cousounis P. Internet peer support for individuals with psychiatric disabilities: a randomized controlled trial. Soc Sci Med. 2011;72(1):54–62.
15. Proudfoot J, Parker G, Manicavasagar V, Hadzi-Pavlovic D, Whitton A, Nicholas J, et al. Effects of adjunctive peer support on perceptions of illness control and understanding in an online psychoeducation program for bipolar disorder: a randomised controlled trial. J Affect Disord. 2012;142(1–3):98–105.
16. Davidson L, Shahar G, Stayner DA, Chinman MJ, Rakfeldt J, Tebes JK. Supported socialization for people with psychiatric disabilities: lessons from a randomized controlled trial. J Community Psychol. 2004;32(4):453–77.
17. Pitt V, Lowe D, Hill S, Prictor M, Hetrick SE, Ryan R, et al. Consumer-providers of care for adult clients of statutory mental health services. Cochrane Database Syst Rev. 2013;2013(3):CD004807.
18. Fuhr DC, Salisbury TT, De Silva MJ, Atif N, van Ginneken N, Rahman A, et al. Effectiveness of peer-delivered interventions for severe mental illness and depression on clinical and psychosocial outcomes: a systematic review and meta-analysis. Soc Psychiatry Psychiatr Epidemiol. 2014;49(11):1691–702.
19. Chinman M, George P, Dougherty RH, Daniels AS, Ghose SS, Swift A, et al. Peer support services for individuals with serious mental illnesses: assessing the evidence. Psychiatr Serv. 2014;65(4):429–41. https://doi.org/10.1176/appi.ps.201300244.
20. Fisher EB, Boothroyd RI, Elstad EA, Hays L, Henes A, Maslow GR, et al. Peer support of complex health behaviors in prevention and disease management with special reference to diabetes: systematic reviews. Clin Diabetes Endocrinol. 2017;3(1):4.
21. Landers GM, Zhou M. An analysis of relationships among peer support, psychiatric hospitalization, and crisis stabilization. Community Ment Health J. 2011;47(1):106–12.
22. Sells D, Davidson L, Jewell C, Falzer P, Rowe M. The treatment relationship in peer-based and regular case management for clients with severe mental illness. Psychiatr Serv. 2006;57(8):1179–84.
23. Jones N, Corrigan PW, James D, Parker J, Larson N. Peer support, self-determination, and treatment engagement: a qualitative investigation. Psychiatr Rehabil J. 2013;36(3):209.
24. Gidugu V, Rogers ES, Harrington S, Maru M, Johnson G, Cohee J, et al. Individual peer support: a qualitative study of mechanisms of its effectiveness. Community Ment Health J. 2015;51(4):445–52.
25. Davidson L, Bellamy C, Guy K, Miller R. Peer support among persons with severe mental illnesses: a review of evidence and experience. World Psychiatry. 2012;11(2):123–8.

26. Festinger L. A theory of social comparison processes. Hum Relat. 1954;7(2):117–40.
27. Bandura A. Social learning theory. Englewood Cliffs: Prentice Hall; 1977.
28. Bandura A. Self-efficacy: the exercise of control. New York: W.H. Freeman; 1997.
29. Dixon LB, Dickerson F, Bellack AS, Bennett M, Dickinson D, Goldberg RW, et al. The 2009 schizophrenia PORT psychosocial treatment recommendations and summary statements. Schizophr Bull. 2009;36(1):48–70.
30. Chien WT, Clifton AV, Zhao S, Lui S. Peer support for people with schizophrenia or other serious mental illness. Cochrane Database Syst Rev. 2019;2019(4):CD010880.
31. Chien W-T, Norman I. The effectiveness and active ingredients of mutual support groups for family caregivers of people with psychotic disorders: a literature review. Int J Nurs Stud. 2009;46(12):1604–23.
32. Chien W-T, Thompson DR, Norman I. Evaluation of a peer-led mutual support group for Chinese families of people with schizophrenia. Am J Community Psychol. 2008;42(1–2):122–34.
33. Chien WT. Effectiveness of psychoeducation and mutual support group program for family caregivers of chinese people with schizophrenia. Open Nurs J. 2008;2:28.
34. Chien WT, Thompson DR. An RCT with three-year follow-up of peer support groups for Chinese families of persons with schizophrenia. Psychiatr Serv. 2013;64(10):997–1005.
35. Castelein S, Mulder PJ, Bruggeman R. Guided peer support groups for schizophrenia: a nursing intervention. Psychiatr Serv. 2008;59(3):326.
36. Castelein S, Bruggeman R, Van Busschbach JT, Van Der Gaag M, Stant A, Knegtering H, et al. The effectiveness of peer support groups in psychosis: a randomized controlled trial. Acta Psychiatr Scand. 2008;118(1):64–72.
37. Boardman G, McCann T, Kerr D. A peer support programme for enhancing adherence to oral antipsychotic medication in consumers with schizophrenia. J Adv Nurs. 2014;70(10):2293–302.
38. Rummel-Kluge C, Stiegler-Kotzor M, Schwarz C, Hansen W-P, Kissling W. Peer-counseling in schizophrenia: patients consult patients. Patient Educ Couns. 2008;70(3):357–62.
39. Dixon LB, Holoshitz Y, Nossel I. Treatment engagement of individuals experiencing mental illness: review and update. World Psychiatry. 2016;15(1):13–20.
40. Pawson R, Greenhalgh T, Harvey G, Walshe K. Realist review-a new method of systematic review designed for complex policy interventions. J Health Serv Res Policy. 2005;10(1_suppl):21–34.
41. Rycroft-Malone J, McCormack B, Hutchinson AM, DeCorby K, Bucknall TK, Kent B, et al. Realist synthesis: illustrating the method for implementation research. Implement Sci. 2012;7(1):33.
42. Jagosh J. Realist synthesis for public health: building an ontologically deep understanding of how programs work, for whom, and in which contexts. Annu Rev Public Health. 2019;40:361.
43. Rogers ES, Swarbrick M. Peer-delivered services: current trends and innovations. Psychiatr Rehabil J. 2016;39(3):193–6.
44. Gillard S, Gibson S, Holley J, Lucock M. Developing a change model for peer worker interventions in mental health services: a qualitative research study. Epidemiol Psychiatr Sci. 2015;24(5):435–45.

Chapter 6
Realist Perspective and Methodology

The research presented in this book is guided by the overarching question: "What applications of peer support utilized in practice are reaching with people with schizophrenia and how are those applications bringing about benefits?" This question was explored through two research activities: (1) a realist review of the literature (an approach designed to advance understanding of *what* works for *whom* in *what circumstances*) and (2) semi-structured in-depth interviews with key informants with expertise in the field of peer support for mental health. These two methods were designed to work together and inform each other and were undertaken in an iterative fashion with the literature review guiding the development of the interview guide and interviewees commenting on the results of the literature review. These two research activities advanced three aims:

Aim 1: Through a realist review of the literature, characterize (a) the ways in which peer support is being used in practice with people diagnosed with schizophrenia and (b) processes by and contexts in which benefits of peer support for people with schizophrenia are achieved.

Aim 2: Through discussion of the results of Aim 1 with experts in the field of peer support for mental health, clarify the findings of the realist review as well as obtain feedback regarding omissions, errors, and refinements.

Aim 3: Through the literature review and expert interviews, identify and explore implementation facilitators, barriers, and key challenges in the field.

These research activities are well positioned to advance an understanding of the theoretical underpinnings of peer support programming for people with schizophrenia, providing specifics about what activities are included in peer support interventions as well as the benefits they are intended to bring about. As peer support is a complex intervention that can be delivered in many different formats, efficacy trials may not always be sufficient to document or test the complexities involved in the intervention to provide explanations of why they work or fail to work. Likewise, systematic reviews and meta-analyses are driven by a hierarchy of methods and prioritize RCTs over other types of evidence. A meta-analysis, which pools results of many efficacy trials, may not fully capture the many complexities in how intervention components are delivered which may impact their demonstrated efficacy. As the research presented here was primarily concerned with these complexities, methods such as these were not appropriate.

M. Evans, *Peer Support Services Reaching People with Schizophrenia*,
https://doi.org/10.1007/978-3-031-29042-8_6

6.1 Realist Perspective Framing This Research

Realism has been advanced as a post-positivist methodological orientation that perceives social change to be neither linear nor haphazard but transformational [1], meaning that social programs change the context in which they are implemented at the macro-, meso-, and microlevels [2]. Realism presumes the existence of an external world in which events are triggered by underlying mechanisms [3]. A realist orientation places a priority on the lessons drawn from practice [3]. Favoring neither qualitative nor quantitative methods, realism is primarily concerned with production of theories of the middle range [1]. A middle range theory is one that is not so abstract that it is disconnected from on-the-ground workings of programs but also not so specific as to only pertain to one program [4]. Situated between positivism and constructivism, realism employs a generative approach to causation [2, 5]. The positivist model, which underlies clinical trials, purports that causality is established when cause X is activated in an experiment and effect Y follows [6]. In contrast, a generative approach infers a causal outcome between two events when one understands the underlying mechanism that connects them and the context in which the relationship occurs [6].

Realism begins with the question: "What is it about a program that works?" [5]. It acknowledges that programs provide resources that are internalized by people exposed to the program, and thus, it is not the intervention in isolation that works or fails to work [5]. Rather, it considers the interaction between context, mechanism, and outcome and thereby can explain examples of success, failure, and various eventualities in between [2]. Mechanisms are defined as the underlying entities, processes, or structures which operate in particular contexts to generate outcomes of interest [7]. Mechanisms are not always visible but can be inferred from the observable data; they are context sensitive; and they generate outcomes [8]. It should be noted that the knowledge generated by realist research should not be thought of as causal in a positivist sense. Rather, realist research aims to generate collective wisdom of the ways in which complex interventions bring about outcomes [1].

The research presented here employs realism as a frame through which to investigate the research question. As peer support interventions are expanding in mental health care, identifying aspects that may be particularly important to their effectiveness in different contexts is warranted. At their core, interventions are theories of change, designed to impact outcomes through specific mechanisms. They may result in different outcomes depending on the contexts in which they are delivered. From the perspectives of policy makers and those responsible for program design and implementation, understanding *what* works for *whom* in *what circumstances* may be more useful than results from a systematic review and meta-analysis that conclude that experimental research to date demonstrates that peer support is effective or ineffective among people with schizophrenia. This research is designed to illuminate the nuanced ways in which peer support is conceptualized and delivered, the myriad ways in which it is intended to provide benefit, and the explanations of how peer support activities might bring about such benefits. In this way, it is focused on creating collective knowledge of the ways in which peer support interventions bring about benefits, especially for people with schizophrenia.

6.2 Research Activity 1: Realist Review of the Literature

6.2.1 Overview of Realist Review Methodology

A realist synthesis, or realist review, applies realist philosophy to the synthesis of findings from primary sources that have a bearing on a single research question or set of questions [2]. It focuses on understanding and unpacking the mechanisms by which an intervention works or fails to work and, thus, provides explanations of how it works as opposed to a judgment of effectiveness [6]. Realist review is particularly well suited to analyzing complex interventions [9], or interventions that are made up of multiple components, consisting mainly of human interactions, which produce outcomes [10]. Human decision-making as well as the context within and beyond the intervention influences the nature of the interactions [10]. The focus in realist reviews is explanatory and not evaluative, aiming to uncover potential mechanisms by which complex interventions bring about their outcomes. Systematic reviews and meta-analyses of randomized controlled trials may answer questions regarding efficacy and effectiveness but would not be appropriate to answer the question of why and how peer support interventions work in aiding mental health recovery. Theory generation and refinement are the fundamental objectives of realist review [6].

6.2.2 Research Aim

The primary aim of the realist review was to investigate the peer support activities being utilized among people with schizophrenia and related disorders and the outcomes these activities are intended to bring about. Furthermore, the review was designed to facilitate a deeper understanding of the contexts in which benefits of peer support are brought forth as well as potential mechanisms linking activity and benefit, allowing for the creation of a theoretical understanding of the ways in which peer support works to generate favorable outcomes among people with schizophrenia and related psychoses. This addressed a documented gap in the literature: the lack of theoretical models underlying PS programs [11–15]. This "theory integrity" strategy also facilitates the discovery of typical weak points or stumbling blocks in the program theory that might account for null or adverse effects [6]. The theoretical constructs identified as important might be measured in future research, and relationships among them explored.

Furthermore, the review sought to provide practical guidance on key issues and challenges in the field, such as facilitators and barriers to successful implementation, establishing peer role definition and differentiation, professionalization of the peer role, and the negotiation of complex interpersonal boundaries between peers and those they support. This secondary aim of the review was to directly inform practice, an important consideration given that the evidence base for peer support has not kept pace with the proliferation of peer programs in the field [16].

The realist review method described in the Realist and Meta-narrative Evidence Synthesis: Evolving Standards (RAMESES) publication standards guided this review. As outlined here, the essential steps in a realist review are as follows: (1) clarifying the scope of the review, (2) articulating the relevant underlying theories, (3) searching for evidence, (4) appraising the evidence, and (5) synthesizing the evidence [2, 17]. Each step is described in detail below. It should be noted that the process through stages was iterative and not linear as it is described for the sake of clarity.

6.2.3 *Stage 1: Clarification of the Scope of Review*

In this stage, the main research activities were identifying the research question, clarifying the purpose of the review, and finding and articulating potential theories underlying the intervention to be tested throughout the review [6]. The preliminary research question identified was as follows: "In its current applications, what benefits are noted for peer support in schizophrenia, what explanations linking applications and benefits are being put forth, and what types of potential application and benefit of peer support are not being included in care and rehabilitation of those with schizophrenia?" To focus the review, an exploratory scoping of the literature in several steps was completed.

6.2.3.1 Review of Systematic Reviews and Meta-Analyses

First, I completed a review of systematic reviews and meta-analyses of peer support interventions for mental health. Five systematic reviews were included in this initial step [12, 13, 18–20]. To integrate and synthesize findings from these reviews, I identified the original articles identified in these systematic reviews and organized them according to a typology that has been used to categorize peer support interventions in diabetes [21, 22]. After searching the reference lists and eliminating duplicates, 42 original papers were identified. Of these, 40 full text articles were located. One paper described an intervention that was aimed at physical health management among people with SMI [23] and, as it did not address specific mental health outcomes, was excluded from further review.

Utilizing the typology set out by Heisler [21, 22], each intervention was classified as belonging to one of the following types: (1) peer coaches or mentors, (2) face-to-face group self-management programs, (3) telephone-based peer support,

(4) Web- and email-based support, and (5) others. The classification of peer coaches or mentors included studies that investigated the effect of peers operating in traditional mental health service roles such as case managers as well as those fulfilling more independent peer support functions. One paper described a multisite trial, which combined results from eight different interventions that spanned different types of peer support [24]. Including the eight programs identified in that paper, a total of 40 unique interventions were described. In addition to the variety of intervention types, studies measured many different outcomes. These were sorted into four categories: (1) recovery-related outcomes, such as empowerment or hope, (2) symptoms and functioning, (3) psychosocial outcomes such as self-efficacy and quality of life, and (4) objective events, such as use of clinical services, hospitalizations, or arrests. Results from this initial step in the exploratory scoping of the literature were used to guide the following steps of the realist review.

6.2.3.2 Refining the Research Question

After this initial exploratory literature search and review, the research question was refined to include the following series of questions intended to guide the realist review:

1. What strategies or activities are the peer supporters employing in identified peer support programs?
2. What outcomes are affected by these strategies and activities?
3. What mechanisms or mediating variables are proposed to link strategies/activities to outcomes?
4. What contexts or settings are associated with benefit?

A defining feature of realist reviews is the identification of the theoretical drivers for the intervention under review, which are then interrogated using the evidence of the review. Through the initial exploratory search of the literature, it became apparent that few evidence sources identify an explicit framework underlying their peer support interventions. One exception was found in Gillard et al. [25]. Through qualitative interviews with peer workers, service users, staff, and managers of 10 different peer support programs, these authors identified that the first step to effective peer support interventions lies in building trusting relationships based on shared lived experience [25]. Through this, peer supporters can act as role models and bridges between consumers and providers [25]. Shared lived experiences and bridging between consumers and providers are likely to impact these potential mediating factors: hope in the future, empowerment, social functioning, self-care, engagement with services, and strength of social networks [25]. Through these mechanisms of action, peer support services are thought to be able to impact downstream outcomes such as increased recovery, well-being, and service use [25]. These proposed theoretical constructs were interrogated with evidence from this review.

Additionally, the conceptual model of peer support developed after the first step of the exploratory literature search was also considered a "candidate theory" to be revised and expanded upon with additional evidence identified through the realist review. The model is presented in Chap. 3 (Fig. 3.1).

6.2.4 Stage 2: Searching for Evidence

Published and grey literature sources were identified by employing a comprehensive search strategy consisting of several steps. First, to identify published literature sources, searches were conducted in several relevant databases: PsycInfo, PubMed, Scopus, CINAHL, CENTRAL, and Web of Science. The following search terms were utilized:

> *Peer support* (Peer-support OR "peer support" OR coach* OR "Community Health Workers"[Mesh] OR "community health worker*" OR "lay health worker*" OR "lay health advisor" OR "natural helper*" OR "peer educator" OR "community health aide" OR "health advocate*" OR "community health promoter" OR "community health representative" OR "outreach worker*" OR "dumas*" OR "embajadores" OR "consejeras" OR "consumer provider*") AND *'Schizophrenia or Serious Mental Illness'* ("Schizophrenia"[Mesh] OR schizophreni* OR "psychosis" OR "SMI" OR "serious mental illness" OR "severe mental illness").

These search terms for the different cognates for peer supporters were adapted from previous literature reviews [20, 26] and revised to include the term "consumer provider," a term frequently used in US mental health services. To capture literature regarding peer support interventions that are delivered to mixed-diagnosis groups, a common strategy identified through the exploratory literature search, the search term "serious mental illness" was included in addition to "schizophrenia" and "psychosis."

Next, a systematic search of the grey literature was undertaken. Dissertations were identified from Networked Digital Library of Theses and Dissertations and ProQuest Dissertations and Theses Global. Clinical trials were identified through the following resources: clinicaltrials.gov, WHO's International Clinical Trials Registry Platform, and NIH Reporter. Conference proceedings were identified through Embase and Scopus. Finally, the websites identified in the Grey Matters checklist were searched to identify relevant health-related literature [27].

Citations identified through the published literature search were downloaded into EndNote [28] and uploaded into Covidence [29]. Duplicates were removed both automatically using EndNote's de-duplication procedure and manually during the abstract screening process. Resources identified through the grey literature search were downloaded and manually entered in EndNote. Titles and abstracts were screened in Covidence.

6.2.5 *Stage 3: Data Extraction*

To inform the strategy for data extraction, an initial review of 20 articles was completed. To mirror the distribution between the published and grey literature resources, 13 of the papers reviewed were identified through the published literature search and the remaining seven through the grey literature search. Through the process of completing this initial review, it became apparent that an adequate data abstraction method required in-depth review of additional literature sources. To accomplish this, the published literature sources were reviewed by publication date starting with the most recent. Each document was interrogated with the following questions: (1) "What peer support approaches are described?" (2) "How are they beneficial?" (3) "Why?" Sections of text that answered any of these questions were coded in Atlas. ti [30]. Additionally, sections of text that discussed a key theme with potential relevance to the field (e.g., stigma, match between peers and those they support, role boundaries, etc.) were also coded. After reviewing each evidence source, a brief description of the paper, any codes added to capture relevant information, and any ideas to organizing results were documented in a research memo.

Through this approach, I developed a codebook of emergent codes. New codes were added throughout the data extraction process on an as-needed basis. The final codebook contained 73 codes. Twenty-seven of the codes identified different types of evidence, including intervention studies, quantitative studies, qualitative studies, literature reviews, registered clinical trials, and commentaries. Integral to the realist review approach, codes captured peer support strategies or activities, potential mechanisms, and measured outcomes, along with whether the findings favored the peer support condition, the control condition, or were equivocal between the two. Several important themes arising from the initial exploratory literature search were also coded in these documents, such as match, implementation facilitators, implementation barriers, and role boundaries. This approach was utilized to extract data from all included published and grey literature sources.

6.2.6 *Stage 4: Data Synthesis and Drawing Conclusions*

Data synthesis occurred simultaneously with data extraction, with information from each new article reviewed being situated within the information gleaned from previous sources. Data analysis was undertaken with an explanatory function in mind: understanding the mechanisms of specific peer support strategies that generate outcomes in particular contexts. Theory building and refinement were the primary goal of this stage of the review. Additionally, data relating to important issues for the field, identified and coded in the data extraction phase, were synthesized to provide summaries of key issues and challenges for the field.

Developing categorization systems to synthesize the data was an iterative process. Initially, studies were organized according to the types of peer intervention described: clinical services provided by peers, psychosocial services provided by peers, and other services or interventions supported by peers. Later, categories for naturally occurring peer support interventions and community health worker (CHW) interventions were added. The approach continued to evolve throughout the data extraction and synthesis phases. An important distinction was illuminated: Some interventions were targeting mental health management, while others focused on physical health management. Due to the potential different strategies employed to address these different, albeit related, phenomena, the analysis of these categories was separated. Thus, one set of results presented relates to peer support interventions focused on mental health management, and another relates to those focused on physical health management. Within interventions focused on mental health, interventions were further categorized based on their relation to clinical services: standalone peer support services with no formal connection to clinical services, peer support services delivered in conjunction with clinical services, and clinical, paraclinical, or case management services delivered by peers.

For each study that described a particular intervention, other contextual factors of the intervention were documented, including format, medium, peer type, role of peer, hosting organization, and target population. These were documented in Excel [31], and frequencies of the contextual factors of included interventions were calculated. Evidence tables documenting the peer support strategies and activities of the described intervention, any potential mechanisms suggested, outcomes measured, and significant findings were created. Through the process of compiling evidence tables, the format of each evidence table was refined to group together like strategies, potential mechanisms, and outcomes.

To achieve Aim 3 and summarize important issues for the field, code reports were created in Atlas.ti for the following codes: stigma, facilitators, barriers, role boundaries, differences between peer and clinical providers, needs of peer supporters, peer contributions to research, peer support training and supervision, guidance or recommendations, and match. These reports enabled evidence synthesis across numerous sources.

6.2.7 Stage 5: Dissemination, Implementation, and Evaluation

The results of the realist review were used to develop the interview guide, which provided a summary of results and prompted stakeholders to provide their expert input into the findings. This book is another of the products of the dissemination stage of the realist review.

6.3 Research Activity 2: Expert Interviews

Semi-structured in-depth interviews with experts in the field of peer support for mental health were conducted to achieve Aims 2 and 3. The primary focus of these interviews was to triangulate the findings from the realist review and adapt them to be of the most utility to important stakeholders. To do so, interview participants were asked to identify any oversights or misrepresentation in the results of the realist review as well as provide their general feedback on themes that have emerged as key issues in the field. Interviews were conducted via Zoom [32] and recorded with consent. Zoom transcripts were generated and finalized by listening to the audio recordings and correcting transcription errors. Transcripts were thematically analyzed [33]. This research was reviewed by the Institutional Review Board at the University of North Carolina at Chapel Hill and deemed exempt (IRB Study #: 21-2887).

6.3.1 Sampling and Recruitment

Interviewees were purposively sampled utilizing a criterion sampling method [34]. The criterion on which interviewees were selected was their expertise in the field of peer support for mental health. Throughout the process of completing the realist review, key people and organizations that are doing considerable work in the field of peer support for mental health were identified. These key stakeholders included leading researchers in the field, advocates, representatives from nonprofit organizations, peer support associations, and government entities. After completing the realist review, a list of 24 potential interviewees was generated, email addresses from publicly available websites were obtained, and recruitment emails were sent. Some interview respondents suggested additional people to interview and provided them with the interviewer's contact information. Further interviews with these experts were conducted when these individuals contacted the interviewer and agreed to participate.

6.3.2 Interview Topics

The interview guide consisted of a series of questions intended to gain the perspectives of expert interviewees on the topics relevant to the realist review, in particular peer support strategies, important outcomes, and potential mechanisms linking activity to benefit. Participants were asked to comment on findings regarding these topics, including any omissions or mischaracterizations. Additionally, participants provided insights into key facilitators and barriers to successful implementation and crucial challenges in the field. Participants provided their thoughts about the most important issues for the field. Finally, participants were asked if there was anything critical to the field that was omitted or misrepresented in the interview.

6.3.3 Data Collection and Analysis

Data collection and analysis occurred simultaneously in an iterative fashion. Interviews were conducted via Zoom and recorded with consent. Upon completion of each interview, field notes from the interview were reviewed and compiled into an outline used to identify emerging themes. Each transcript generated by Zoom was reviewed and corrected as needed. Each transcript was anonymized and assigned a unique identifier, and responses to each interview question were compiled across all interviews. A file linking the interviewee names and their unique identifiers was maintained in a secure, password-protected location.

Transcripts were first read after interviews occurred and then, on subsequent reads, were thematically analyzed using deductive and inductive codes [33]. Deductive codes were derived from the key issues presented and expanded upon in the interviews (e.g., professionalization, boundaries, etc.). Additionally, codes were developed to identify whether interviewees agreed with realist review findings, disagreed with realist review findings, or noted omissions in the realist review findings. Finally, two inductive codes were generated during the analysis process: peer support infrastructure and payment. An analytic matrix was used to help reduce and synthesize the qualitative data and identify emergent themes. Results are presented in the following two chapters.

References

1. Pawson R. Evidence-based policy: a realist perspective. London: Sage; 2006.
2. Wong G, Greenhalgh T, Westhorp G, Buckingham J, Pawson R. RAMESES publication standards: realist syntheses. BMC Med. 2013;11(1):21.
3. Mark MM, Henry GT, Julnes G, Mark M, Henry G. Evaluation: an integrated framework for understanding. Guiding, and improving policies and programs. San Francisco: Jossey-Bass; 2000.
4. Jagosh J. Realist synthesis for public health: building an ontologically deep understanding of how programs work, for whom, and in which contexts. Annu Rev Public Health. 2019;40:361–72.
5. Popay J. Moving beyond effectiveness in evidence synthesis: methodological issues in the synthesis of diverse sources of evidence. London: National Institute for Health and Clinical Excellence; 2006.
6. Pawson R, Greenhalgh T, Harvey G, Walshe K. Realist review – a new method of systematic review designed for complex policy interventions. J Health Serv Res Policy. 2005;10(1_suppl):21–34.
7. Wong G, Westhorp G, Pawson R, Greenhalgh T. Realist synthesis. RAMESES training materials. London: The RAMESES Project; 2013.
8. Astbury B, Leeuw FL. Unpacking black boxes: mechanisms and theory building in evaluation. Am J Eval. 2010;31(3):363–81.
9. Rycroft-Malone J, McCormack B, Hutchinson AM, DeCorby K, Bucknall TK, Kent B, et al. Realist synthesis: illustrating the method for implementation research. Implement Sci. 2012;7(1):33.

10. Wong G. The internet in medical education: a worked example of a realist review. In: Synthesizing qualitative research: choosing the right approach. Chichester: Wiley; 2011. p. 83–112.
11. Bellamy C, Schmutte T, Davidson L. An update on the growing evidence base for peer support. Ment Health Soc Incl. 2017;21(3):161–7.
12. Pitt V, Lowe D, Hill S, Prictor M, Hetrick SE, Ryan R, et al. Consumer-providers of care for adult clients of statutory mental health services. Cochrane Database Syst Rev. 2013;2013(3):CD004807.
13. Lloyd-Evans B, Mayo-Wilson E, Harrison B, Istead H, Brown E, Pilling S, et al. A systematic review and meta-analysis of randomised controlled trials of peer support for people with severe mental illness. BMC Psychiatry. 2014;14(1):39.
14. Evans M, Barker H, Peddireddy S, Zhang A, Luu S, Qian Y, et al. Peer-delivered services and peer support reaching people with schizophrenia: a scoping review. Int J Ment Health. 2021:1–23. https://doi.org/10.1080/00207411.2021.1975441.
15. Davidson L, Chinman M, Sells D, Rowe M. Peer support among adults with serious mental illness: a report from the field. Schizophr Bull. 2006;32(3):443–50.
16. Davidson L. Peer support: coming of age of and/or miles to go before we sleep? An introduction. J Behav Health Serv Res. 2015;42(1):96–9.
17. Wong G, Westhorp G, Manzano A, Greenhalgh J, Jagosh J, Greenhalgh T. RAMESES II reporting standards for realist evaluations. BMC Med. 2016;14(1):96.
18. Fuhr DC, Salisbury TT, De Silva MJ, Atif N, van Ginneken N, Rahman A, et al. Effectiveness of peer-delivered interventions for severe mental illness and depression on clinical and psychosocial outcomes: a systematic review and meta-analysis. Soc Psychiatry Psychiatr Epidemiol. 2014;49(11):1691–702.
19. Chinman M, George P, Dougherty RH, Daniels AS, Ghose SS, Swift A, et al. Peer support services for individuals with serious mental illnesses: assessing the evidence. Psychiatr Serv. 2014;65(4):429–41. https://doi.org/10.1176/appi.ps.201300244.
20. Fisher EB, Boothroyd RI, Elstad EA, Hays L, Henes A, Maslow GR, et al. Peer support of complex health behaviors in prevention and disease management with special reference to diabetes: systematic reviews. Clin Diabetes Endocrinol. 2017;3(1):4.
21. Heisler M. Different models to mobilize peer support to improve diabetes self-management and clinical outcomes: evidence, logistics, evaluation considerations and needs for future research. Fam Pract. 2009;27(suppl_1):i23–32.
22. Heisler M. Overview of peer support models to improve diabetes self-management and clinical outcomes. Diabetes Spectr. 2007;20(4):214–21.
23. Druss BG, Zhao L, Silke A, Bona JR, Fricks L, Jenkins-Tucker S, et al. The Health and Recovery Peer (HARP) Program: a peer-led intervention to improve medical self-management for persons with serious mental illness. Schizophr Res. 2010;118(1–3):264–70.
24. Rogers ES, Teague GB, Lichenstein C, Campbell J, Lyass A, Chen R, et al. Effects of participation in consumer-operated service programs on both personal and organizationally mediated empowerment: results of multisite study. J Rehabil Res Dev. 2007;44:785–800.
25. Gillard S, Gibson S, Holley J, Lucock M. Developing a change model for peer worker interventions in mental health services: a qualitative research study. Epidemiol Psychiatr Sci. 2015;24(5):435–45.
26. Kowitt SD, Ellis KR, Carlisle V, Bhushan NL, Black KZ, Brodar K, et al. Peer support opportunities across the cancer care continuum: a systematic scoping review of recent peer-reviewed literature. Support Care Cancer. 2019;27(1):97–108.
27. Grey matters: a practical tool for searching health-related literature. https://www.cadth.ca/resources/finding-evidence (2018). Accessed, May 29, 2020.
28. The EndNote Team. EndNote. Philadelphia: Clarivate; 2013.
29. Covidence. Melbourne: Veritas Health Innovation; 2020.
30. ATLAS.ti Scientific Software Development GmbH. Atlas.ti: The Qualitative Data Analysis & Research Software. 8.4.5 ed2020.

31. Microsoft Corporation. Microsoft Excel. 2018.
32. ZVC Inc. Security guide. Zoom Video Communications Inc. 2016.
33. Boyatzis RE. Transforming qualitative information: thematic analysis and code development. London: Sage; 1998.
34. Patton MQ. Qualitative research and evaluation methods. Thousand Oakes: Sage; 2002.

Chapter 7
Diversity in Programmatic Features, Peer Support Strategies, Potential Mechanisms, and Outcomes

To best design peer support programs to meet the needs of their intended recipients, it is imperative that we better understand the diverse components that make up these interventions. This chapter presents the results of the realist review which intended to provide such an understanding. First, general results from an exploratory scoping of the literature are presented, followed by detailed results of the realist review. To organize the realist review results, peer interventions were first classified by the focus of the intervention: mental health or physical health. Then, mental health-focused peer support interventions were further classified into the subcategories standalone peer support services, peer support provided in conjunction with clinical services, and peers delivering clinical, paraclinical, or case management services. Contextual and programmatic features, peer support strategies, potential mechanisms, and hypothesized and measured outcomes are presented for each intervention category. Significant findings favoring peer support are highlighted and discussed. Finally, the refinement of the results based on information gained through the key informant interviews is presented.

7.1 Preliminary Findings from Exploratory Scoping of the Literature

Preliminary results from the exploratory scoping of the literature, a review of reviews, indicated that a variety of peer support interventions have been shown to have positive effects on diverse outcomes among people with various mental health diagnoses. However, there are also many instances of null findings. Thirty-nine articles were included in this step of the review [1–39]. Results illuminated areas in which the evidence of the effectiveness of peer support is strong. Of note, group peer support interventions showed significant positive effects on recovery outcomes in all reviewed trials of this intervention type. Most of the group peer support studies also

M. Evans, *Peer Support Services Reaching People with Schizophrenia*, https://doi.org/10.1007/978-3-031-29042-8_7

found significant positive effects on psychosocial outcomes. Additionally, the inclusion of a peer support relationship was shown to increase participants' engagement with Web- and email-based programs. There is some evidence that the services of peer coaches or mentors have positive impacts on varied psychosocial outcomes as well as objective events such as service use and rates of hospitalization.

Additionally, results from this review elucidated areas where evidence of effectiveness is lacking. The few Web- and email-based peer support interventions reviewed had no significant positive effects on recovery or psychosocial outcomes. Likewise, the telephone-based peer support programs had no documented positive effects on psychosocial outcomes except for positive perceptions of the peer support provided. The small number of trials classified into these two groups in this review may account for these null findings, or it may be that peer support interventions provided face-to-face are more potent and effective than their remote counterparts.

From these results, it appears that most of the evidence of peer support is drawn from trials investigating the effectiveness of peer coaches and mentors followed by trials investigating face-to-face peer support groups. Telephone-, Web- and email-based peer support for mental health conditions are much less represented in the published literature. Psychosocial outcomes were much more commonly measured than symptoms or functioning. However, many of the researchers synthesizing the evidence chose to focus on documented effects of peer support on symptoms and objectively measured events, such as acute care utilization. This review was useful in that it teased apart some of the complexities of the ways in which peer support is delivered and its effects measured.

None of the identified studies proposed a theoretical or conceptual model of how the described peer support intervention was intended to work to change outcomes, nor did the authors measure any potential mediators or mechanisms. This lack of theoretical rationale makes it difficult to understand how and why peer support interventions are designed to work and makes compiling evidence from multiple trials difficult. Research would benefit from change models hypothesizing and testing how the specific peer support activities might affect outcomes and through what potential mediators these changes might take place. It may be that some measured psychosocial outcomes, such as attitudes, knowledge, and intentions, are better conceptualized as mediators between peer support activities and more distal outcomes such as symptoms, functioning, quality of life, and use of acute care services. Additionally, recovery-related outcomes might be conceptualized both as outcomes in themselves, as well as potential mediators linking peer support activities, and more distal outcomes such as symptoms, functioning, or service use.

7.2 Overview of Findings from Realist Review

7.2.1 Description of Published and Grey Literature Sources Reviewed

Initially, there were 776 citations identified through both the published (n = 644) and grey literature (n = 132) searches. After removing duplicates, 671 citations remained. From these, 275 sources were deemed irrelevant during title and abstract

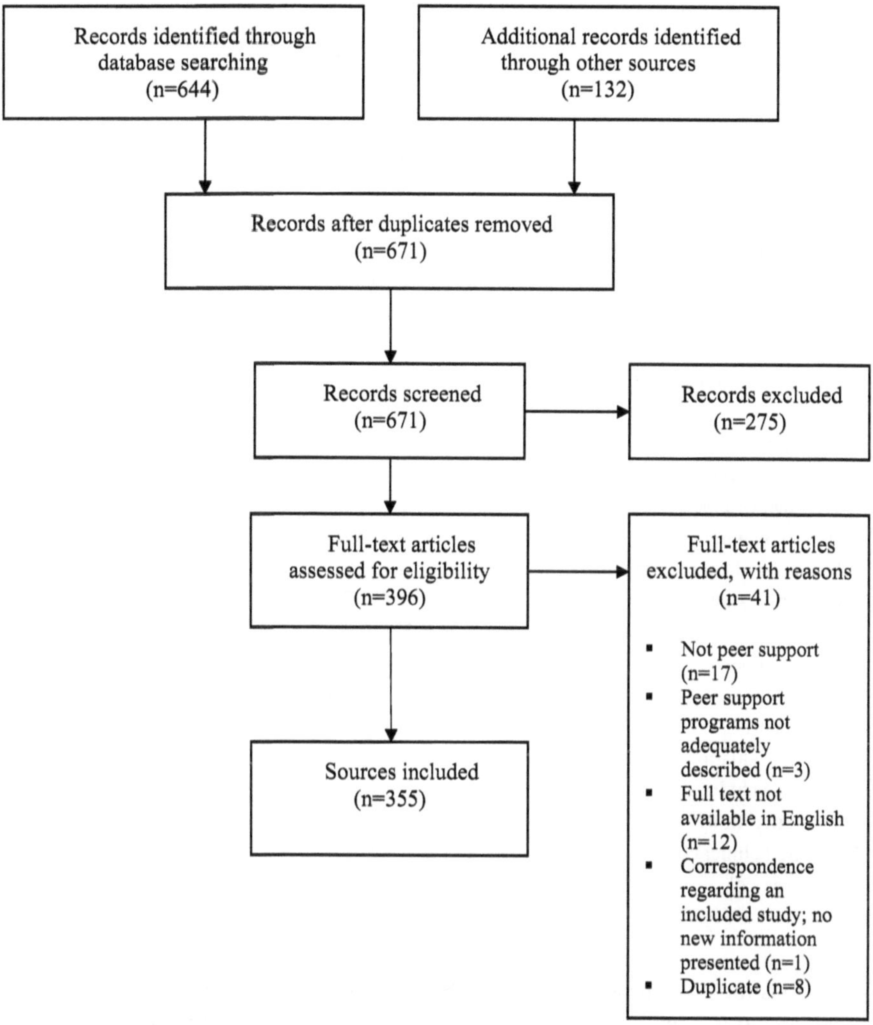

Fig. 7.1 PRISMA diagram

screening, leaving a total of 396 sources for full-text review. Forty-one of those were excluded after full-text review, resulting in a final sample size of 355 published and grey literature sources. The PRISMA diagram presented in Fig. 7.1 documents the disposition of articles at each stage of review.

Table 7.1 presents the type and distribution of all evidence sources reviewed. Most common were literature reviews (12%), intervention studies (11%), qualitative studies (10%), registered clinical trials (10%), and commentaries (10%). Quantitative studies (5%), dissertations and theses (5%), mixed methods studies (5%), feasibility studies (5%), study protocols (4%), program descriptions or development papers (4%), government-funded research reports (4%), and guidance manuals (3%) were also represented. One hundred and thirty-four sources (38%) focused specifically on schizophrenia or psychosis, while the remaining 221 (62%) focused

Table 7.1 Type of evidence reviewed

Type of evidence	*N* (percentage)
Book	3 (0.8%)
Book chapter	8 (2.3%)
Business case analysis	1 (0.3%)
Clinical guideline	4 (1.1%)
Commentary	34 (9.6%)
Commentary with first-person account	2 (0.6%)
Conference abstract	2 (0.6%)
Conference proceedings	3 (0.8%)
Course materials	1 (0.3%)
Development paper/program description	15 (4.2%)
Dissertation or thesis	18 (5.1%)
Feasibility study	17 (4.8%)
First-person account	9 (2.5%)
Government-funded research report	15 (4.2%)
Guidance manual	11 (3.1%)
Information sheet for consumers	2 (0.6%)
Intervention study	38 (10.7%)
Literature review	42 (11.8%)
Mixed methods study	16 (4.5%)
News article	6 (1.7%)
Policy report	2 (0.6%)
Program evaluation	2 (0.6%)
Qualitative study	35 (9.9%)
Quantitative study	19 (5.4%)
Registered clinical trial	35 (9.9%)
Study protocol	13 (3.7%)
Theoretical article	2 (0.6%)

on serious mental illness as a category or on assorted mental health problems. One hundred and fifty unique programs or interventions were described in 171 sources. Some sources provided details for more than one program, while other programs were described in several publications. Other sources did not describe specific programs or interventions, but provided insights on other important factors, such as implementation facilitators, barriers, or key challenges for the field.

7.2.2 *Contexts, Peer Support Strategies, Potential Mechanisms, and Outcomes*

7.2.2.1 Contextual and Programmatic Features

The 150 programs varied considerably on contextual and programmatic features including intervention format, intervention medium, role of the peer(s), focus of the intervention, hosting organization, and target population. Descriptive statistics of

Table 7.2 Contextual and programmatic features of all peer support interventions

Intervention characteristic	*N* (percentage)
Focus of intervention	
Physical health and wellness	14 (9%)
Mental health and wellness	135 (90%)
Hybrid	1 (1%)
Format	
Individual	51 (34%)
Group	64 (43%)
Hybrid	30 (21%)
Not specified	5 (3%)
Medium	
In person	121 (81%)
Online	9 (6%)
Telephone	5 (3%)
Hybrid	9 (6%)
Not specified	6 (4%)
Peer type	
Trained paid peer staff	80 (53%)
Trained volunteers	10 (7%)
Mutual support	49 (33%)
Not specified	11 (7%)
Role of peer	
Peer led	65 (43%)
Peer co-led with professional	38 (25%)
Professionally led with express encouragement of mutual support among participants	13 (9%)
Mutual support with no identified supporter	20 (13%)
Flexible	9 (6%)
Not specified	5 (3%)
Hosting organization	
Healthcare organization	4 (3%)
Behavioral healthcare organization	72 (48%)
Consumer-operated service organization	28 (19%)
Research project	27 (18%)
Other	16 (11%)
Not specified	3 (2%)
Target population	
People with SMI	104 (69%)
People with schizophrenia	45 (30%)
Not specified	1 (1%)

contextual and programmatic features are presented in Table 7.2. Intervention formats included individual (one-to-one) peer support and services, group peer support interventions, and programs that included a combination of individual and group approaches. Programs were delivered in person, via telephone, online, or in some combination of these mediums through a variety of hosting organizations, including physical healthcare organizations, behavioral or mental healthcare organizations, research projects, and peer-run organizations. Peers led interventions independently in 43% of interventions and co-led with clinicians in another 25%. Other programs (13%) consisted of mutual support without an identified supporter. A well-known example of this type of approach is Alcoholics Anonymous, where people come together and support each other in dealing with a common problem, but there is no identified group leader and relationships are egalitarian. Furthermore, some programs described peer support as taking place in clinician-led group therapy. Interventions of this type were included only if they explicitly described the encouragement of mutual support among participants as a core goal of the program.

The primary focus of the peer program also varied. Fourteen programs (9%) focused primarily on improving physical health problems for people with schizophrenia or other serious mental illnesses, 135 (90%) focused primarily on improving mental health among these populations, and one (1%) focused equally on both physical and mental health outcomes. Another two focused largely on other issues (parenting, using the internet to locate information and services) and, thus, were not included in these results. Results of the physical health-focused interventions and the mental health-focused interventions are presented separately; however, it should be noted that there is indeed an important relationship between physical and mental health. Most programs (69%) were intended for populations with any serious mental illness, while only 30% focused on people with schizophrenia or psychosis specifically.

Figure 7.2 presents an overview of the detailed peer support strategies, potential mechanisms, and outcomes discussed below.

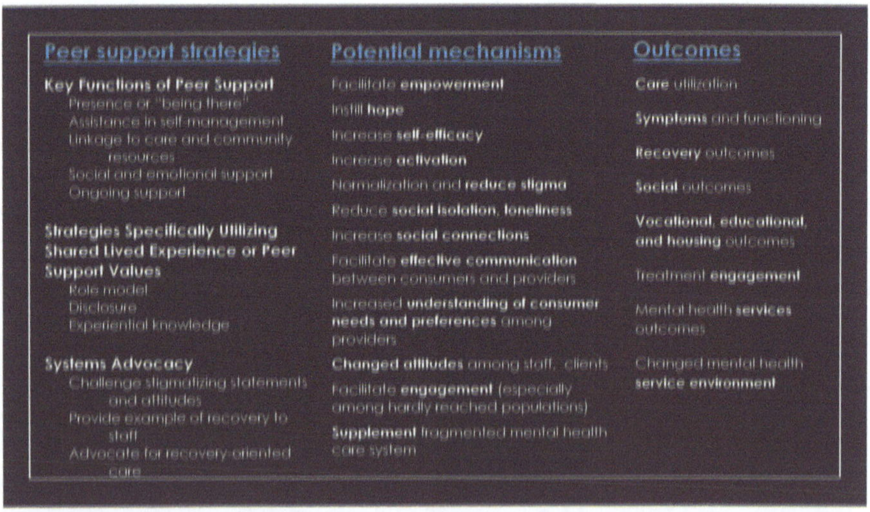

Fig. 7.2 Common peer support strategies, mechanisms, and outcomes of mental health-focused peer support programs

7.2.2.2 Peer Support Strategies

Peer support strategies identified through the realist review included each of the five key functions of peer support described in Chap. 2. The strategies described in the reviewed literature fit well with these key functions, with some clarifications and expansions of definitions. "Being there" comprised social activities and explicit focus on companionship. Assistance in self-management of mental health encompassed different strategies than assistance in self-management of physical health conditions and included a wide variety of strategies such as psychoeducation, developing coping skills, goal setting, action planning, and problem solving. Here, linkage to clinical care and community resources was defined liberally, involving referrals, assistance in navigating care and service systems, and liaising between consumers and providers. In addition, peer advocacy and encouragement of self-advocacy for the individual's care needs and preferences with healthcare providers and social services agencies were included as part of this key function. Social and emotional support included emotional, informational, instrumental, and appraisal support. Ongoing care was operationalized as support that lasts at least 3 months, services that provide between-session check-ins, care that is available outside of normal business hours, or a stepped care design through which support increases or decreases over time according to individual needs.

In addition to the key functions, some strategies identified in the literature explicitly utilized shared lived experience or were grounded in peer support values. These strategies included role modeling recovery, instilling hope by providing a living example of recovery, giving suggestions grounded in experiential knowledge, and developing nonhierarchical relationships. These might be characterized as the "essence" of peer support. While the key functions could, in theory, be provided by anyone, these strategies are specifically using the peers' lived experience as a basis for providing support. Finally, some sources identified a function of peer support that occurs in clinical and community mental health spaces—influencing and transforming care systems to be more recovery oriented. This might happen through peers' actions such as by challenging stigmatizing language used by staff, identifying discriminatory organizational policies, or providing an example of recovery to staff and changing their attitudes on what is possible for people with mental illnesses.

7.2.2.3 Potential Mechanisms

Potential mechanisms identified fell along different levels of the socioecological model. On the individual level, peer support was suggested to facilitate empowerment, instill hope, increase self-efficacy to manage mental illness, increase activation, and reduce self-stigma. On an interpersonal level, peer support may reduce loneliness and social isolation and increase social relationships. It can also improve communication between individuals and their healthcare providers, helping providers to better understand the needs and preferences of the individuals they serve. On an organizational level, peers may bring about organizational change within mental healthcare systems. On the community and societal levels, the very existence of peer support specialists can increase general awareness of mental health and recovery, normalize mental illness, and reduce stigma.

7.2.2.4 Outcomes

Outcomes measured in the literature included those more clinical in nature, such as care utilization, especially utilization of acute care; symptoms and functioning; and treatment engagement or adherence. In addition to these clinical outcomes, many studies focused on recovery outcomes, including quality of life, empowerment, and self-rated recovery. Some measured social outcomes, such as level of social support, content of social networks, or social functioning. Vocational, educational, and housing outcomes were infrequently measured. Finally, mental health services outcomes, such as satisfaction with care and number of met and unmet care needs, were also represented in the literature.

To avoid the flattening effect of grouping all interventions together, results of this review are presented in two categories: programs focused on improving physical health and those focused on improving mental health. Results of programs focused on mental health are divided into three subcategories: standalone peer support services, peer support provided in conjunction with clinical services, and peers delivering clinical, paraclinical, or case management services. Table 7.3 provides a comparison of the proportion of programs of each type reporting each of the identified peer support strategies, potential mechanisms, and hypothesized outcomes. Figure 7.3 depicts the comparison of the proportion of peer support strategies utilized within each program category.

7.3 Peer Interventions Focused on Improving Physical Health among People with SMI

7.3.1 Contextual and Programmatic Features

Fourteen unique interventions focused on improving physical health outcomes among people with schizophrenia or SMI. These programs were described in 24 sources. Contextual and programmatic features of these are presented in Table 7.4. Most (43%) were delivered to individuals, 36% in group format, and the remaining 21% in a combination of individual and group formats. The most common mode of intervention was in person (64%), and most programs (71%) were delivered by trained peer staff. Peer staff were involved in leading most of the described interventions, independently in half of the programs and in conjunction with a professional in another 36%. Fourteen percent were mutual support interventions where there

Table 7.3 Proportional comparison of peer support strategies, potential mechanisms, and hypothesized outcomes by program type

		Mental health focused		
	Physical health focused	Standalone peer programs	Peer support provided in conjunction with clinical care	Clinical, paraclinical or case management services provided by peers
	(n = 14)	(n = 43)	(n = 76)	(n = 16)
Peer support strategies				
"Being there"	14%	51%	42%	6%
Assistance in self-management	71%	35%	57%	38%
Linkage to clinical care and community resources	50%	19%	43%	44%
Social and emotional support	43%	35%	39%	31%
Ongoing support	71%	21%	42%	19%
Strategies specifically utilizing shared lived experience	36%	33%	45%	69%
Systems advocacy	NA	NA	9%	25%
	Physical health	**Standalone PS**	**PS in conjunction with clinical**	**Clinical, paraclinical, or CM**
Potential mechanisms				
Facilitate empowerment	7%	26%	17%	25%
Instill hope	14%	16%	25%	50%
Increased activation	0%	2%	7%	6%
Increased self-efficacy for self-management	36%	7%	13%	0%
Normalization and reduced stigma	14%	33%	30%	19%
Reduced loneliness and social isolation	0%	19%	14%	0%
Increased social connections	7%	21%	22%	0%
Facilitate effective communication between individuals and healthcare providers	0%	0%	4%	0%
Better understanding of individual wants and needs among healthcare providers	0%	0%	4%	31%
Changed attitudes among staff and clients	0%	0%	8%	25%

(continued)

Table 7.3 (continued)

		Mental health focused		
	Physical health focused	Standalone peer programs	Peer support provided in conjunction with clinical care	Clinical, paraclinical or case management services provided by peers
	(n = 14)	(n = 43)	(n = 76)	(n = 16)
Facilitate engagement	21%	0%	17%	25%
Supplement fragmented mental health system	0%	0%	12%	13%
Hypothesized outcomes				
Care utilization	28%	9%	30%	38%
Mental health symptoms and functioning	0%	9%	33%	38%
Recovery outcomes	36%	14%	39%	38%
Social outcomes	0%	2%	28%	19%
Vocational and educational outcomes	0%	0%	3%	13%
Mental health treatment engagement and adherence	0%	2%	17%	13%
Mental health services outcomes	0%	2%	18%	38%
Changed mental health service environment	0%	0%	5%	13%
Housing outcomes	7%	0%	1%	19%
Substance use	0%	0%	7%	13%
Improved physical health outcomes	86%	0%	0%	0%
Improved health behaviors	57%	0%	0%	0%

was no identified "supporter" and "supported," but rather a group of participants providing support to one another. Research projects not housed within a healthcare facility were the most common site of intervention. The vast majority (93%) of these interventions were intended for people with SMI.

7.3.1.1 Peer Support Strategies

The five key functions were each represented in at least two of the physical health peer programs (14%). "Being there" was the least represented. Perhaps it was not thought to require mention by all authors, especially since the focus was on physical health promotion. Seventy-one percent of programs mentioned assistance in physical health self-management, including strategies such as psychoeducation [40], self-monitoring [41], goal setting [40, 41], and problem-solving [40–42]. Linkage

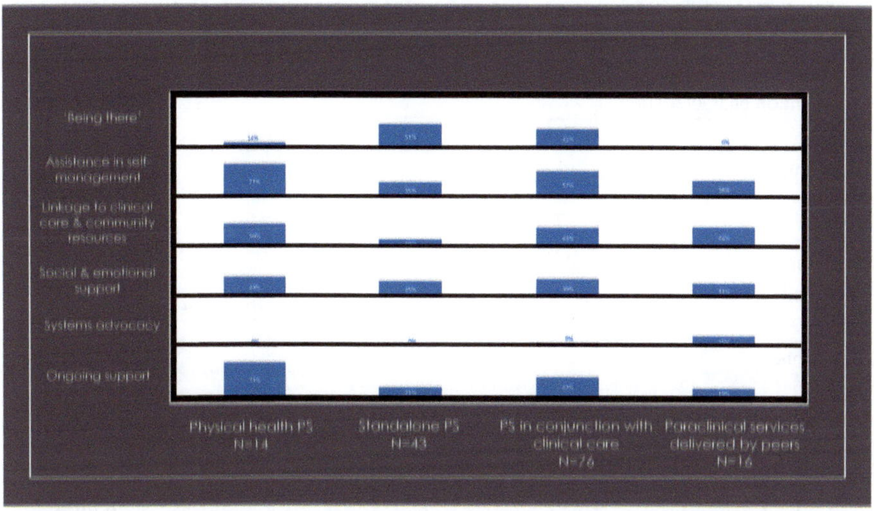

Fig. 7.3 Proportion of programs in each category reporting each peer support strategy

to clinical care or community resources was mentioned by half of the programs, including linking to care [43, 44], peer assistance in navigating care systems [43, 45–48], and working to improve patient-provider communication [46]. Social and emotional support was mentioned in 43% of programs, including emotional, appraisal, informational, and instrumental support [49, 50]. Ongoing support was described in 71% of programs, with 57% lasting at least 3 months [42, 47, 48, 50–55]. Twenty-one percent included check-ins between sessions [41, 44, 49], and 29% described a stepped care design [47, 48, 52, 56]. Only 36% of programs described a strategy that explicitly utilized shared lived experience, such as peers sharing their own experiences, successes, and challenges with health behavior change [46, 49, 51, 53, 57] and acting as role models [41].

7.3.1.2 Potential Mechanisms

Thirteen different mechanisms were proposed by the sources describing physical health interventions. Most common was increasing self-efficacy for health behavior change, mentioned in 36% of programs, followed by promoting engagement in health programming (21%). Normalization of health issues among people with mental health disorders, instilling hope, and increasing peer support for health behavior change were each mentioned by two programs (14%). The remaining proposed mechanisms were each described in one program: facilitating empowerment, enhancing credibility of health-related information, providing opportunities for observational learning, developing shared norms, increasing social relationships, facilitating nonhierarchical relationships, building a mutual learning environment between peer and clinical providers, and reducing distress.

Table 7.4 Contextual and programmatic features of physical health peer support interventions for people with serious mental illnesses

Intervention characteristic	*N* (percentage)
Format	
Individual	6 (43%)
Group	5 (36%)
Hybrid	3 (21%)
Medium	
In person	9 (64%)
Online	0 (0%)
Telephone	1 (7%)
Hybrid	3 (21%)
Not specified	1 (7%)
Peer type	
Trained paid peer staff	10 (71%)
Trained volunteers	0 (0%)
Mutual support	2 (14%)
Not specified	2 (14%)
Role of peer	
Peer led	7 (50%)
Peer co-led with professional	5 (36%)
Professionally led with express encouragement of mutual support among participants	0 (0%)
Mutual support with no identified supporter	2 (14%)
Flexible	0 (0%)
Hosting organization	
Healthcare organization	3 (21%)
Behavioral healthcare organization	5 (36%)
Consumer-operated service organization	0 (0%)
Research project	6 (43%)
Target population	
People with SMI	13 (93%)
People with schizophrenia	1 (7%)

7.3.1.3 Outcomes Measured

Most studies (86%) measured or planned to measure health outcomes, including change in fitness [41, 50, 52, 54, 56], weight [47, 50–52, 55, 56, 58, 59], body mass index [51, 55, 56, 59], hemoglobin A1c [40, 56], cholesterol [52, 56], blood pressure [41, 56], waist circumference [41, 50, 56, 58], bodily pain [48], and physical functioning [41, 53, 58]. Additionally, 57% of studies were interested in health behavior change, such as increasing physical activity [42, 44, 50, 54, 56, 58], improving dietary habits [44, 56, 58], tobacco cessation [53], use of psychiatric medications [53], and substance use [53]. Twenty-one percent of programs measured some aspect of engagement in healthcare, including number of appointments scheduled and attended [45], receiving a physical health screening [46], accessing a general practitioner [46], and improved health literacy [46]. Thirty-six percent of programs measured an aspect of quality of life or well-being [46, 47, 53, 58] and another 36% measured mental health or recovery-related outcomes [47, 50, 53, 56]. The following outcomes were represented in one intervention each: increased goal setting relating to a healthy lifestyle [46], self-management attitudes [48], satisfaction with primary care provider [43, 48], hospitalization [53], and housing status [53].

7.3.1.4 Significant Findings

With regard to weight loss and reduction in body mass index, two programs reported significant results favoring the peer intervention. In one pilot study of a peer group lifestyle intervention with mobile health (mHealth) and social media features, most (72%) of the participants lost weight and 28% achieved a clinically significant weight loss [51]. Weight loss was statistically significant, as was reduction in BMI [51]. In an RCT, participants in an online weight loss program with telephone peer coaching lost an average of 6 pounds over 6 months, while participants in an in-person weight loss program led by a master's level clinician did not lose any weight nor did participants in the treatment as usual condition [55]. In this study, participants who met the criteria for obesity at baseline were also significantly more likely to lose 5% of their body weight in the online weight loss program with peer coaching condition than the in-person, clinician-led weight loss program [55]. In a secondary analysis of data from this trial, significant results favoring the peer intervention compared to usual care were reported for physical activity outcomes (total metabolic-equivalent expenditure (MET) minutes and vigorous MET minutes) [42].

The "Bridge," a peer-delivered health navigator intervention, was effective in increasing visits to, preference for, and relationship quality with routine care providers compared to a waitlist control group [48]. Significant findings were also reported for reduced bodily pain and increased detection of chronic diseases [48]. A further iteration of this program, which included the use of an electronic personal health record, was pilot tested with a group of individuals with SMI who were experiencing housing instability [43]. This study reported significant findings favoring the peer intervention compared to a waitlist control group, including a greater increase in visits to a routine care provider, more health screenings, and an improved relationship with their primary care provider [43]. Furthermore, communication with doctors improved significantly for intervention participants [43].

Another health navigator intervention, a yearlong program intended to increase engagement in primary care among African Americans with SMI who were unhoused, reported significantly more scheduled and achieved appointments among intervention participants than controls [45]. These gains were achieved during the middle 6 months of the program and maintained over the final 3 months [45]. Finally, in a conference abstract from the first Asia Pacific Conference on Integrated

Care, it was reported that receiving support from health peer support workers was associated with increased physical health screening, treatment for comorbidities, health literacy, and healthy lifestyle goal setting [46]. It is worth noting that these findings are from studies focused on people with SMI in general and not specifically on people diagnosed with schizophrenia or a related psychotic disorder.

7.3.1.5 Summary

To generalize, peer-delivered physical health interventions for people with SMI generally assisted in self-management of physical health, linked to clinical care and community resources, and provided ongoing support. Through these activities, they were able to achieve improved physical health outcomes, improved health behaviors, and increased utilization of and engagement in routine health care. These changes were most often hypothesized to be achieved through increasing self-efficacy and promoting engagement in health programming. Full details of these interventions are provided in Table 7.5.

7.4 Peer Interventions Focused on Improving Mental Health

One hundred and thirty-five unique interventions focused on improving mental health were described in 152 evidence sources. To differentiate between many different intervention styles, here peer interventions are defined in relation to their complementarity to clinical services. In some interventions, peer support was provided without any links to or requirements of participating in clinical services. These were classified as standalone peer support services. Another group of programs included at least one peer support component that was designed to be complementary to clinical services. Programs of this type were classified as peer support in conjunction with clinical services. Finally, some interventions described peers delivering services that were initially designed to be delivered by clinical or case management staff, such as case management services, vocational services, or peers as part of ACT teams. Interventions that fit this description were categorized as clinical, paraclinical, or case management services delivered by peers. In some respects, these categorizations resemble the work roles delineated by Moll and colleagues, in which peer workers described their role as supplementary, complementary, or alternative to non-peer clinical staff [60]. Results are presented accordingly.

7.4.1 Standalone Peer Support Services

The types of programs included in this categorization included mutual support groups [61–75], alternatives to inpatient hospitalization [70, 72, 76, 77], drop-in centers and clubhouses [78–80], and online support [28, 71, 81–85]. The mutual support groups described included Hearing Voices Network groups [61–69], an

Table 7.5 Strategies, mechanisms, and outcomes of physical health-focused peer interventions ($n = 14$ programs)

Peer support strategies		
Strategy	**Percentage reporting**	**Examples**
"Being there" (e.g., socialization, companionship, conversation, validation)	14%	Foster a sense of comfort through positive attitude and non-judgmental approach to the work
		Group activities and working toward group goals
Assistance in physical health self-management (e.g., action planning, teaching self-management skills, psychoeducation, problem-solving)	71%	Provide feedback on participants' food logs
		Group weight management and physical activity sessions
		Illness self-management training
		Self-monitoring
		Goal setting
		Problem-solving
		Assessment and planning
		Cognitive-behavioral strategies to support behavior change
		Behavior self-management regarding healthcare
		Specific physical activity suggestions
		Individualized follow-up
		Psychoeducation (regarding stigma, communication with providers, nutrition, monitoring for diabetes and SMI complications, action planning to avoid relapse, etc.)
		Behavioral modeling
		Peer coaching

(continued)

Table 7.5 (continued)

Linkage to clinical care and community resources (e.g., act as liaison between providers and patients, facilitate access to community resources, advocate for consumers with providers, promote engagement in treatment)	50%	Coordinated linkages
		Extend treatment team by engaging and supporting consumers who might not have participated in a program delivered solely by clinicians
		Peer navigation of health services
		Assist care coordinators to increase rate of physical health screening
		Assist consumers to access healthy lifestyle activities and clinical services
		Improve meaningful communication and consumer connection to the treating team
		Peers as part of clinical team in health homes
		Accompany participants to healthcare appointments and follow-up
		Assess community diet and activity resources and develop strategies to address diet and PA needs
		Teaches participants skills to improve healthcare access and use
		Incorporated use of electronic personal health record; navigators had access to their consumers' data
Social and emotional support (e.g., provide emotional support, provide instrumental support, provide informational support)	43%	Facilitate emotional support for health behavior change (e.g., praise and encouragement)
		Facilitate appraisal support for health behavior change (e.g., feedback and social comparison)
		Facilitate informational support for health behavior change (e.g., advice and suggestions)
		Provide instrumental support for health behavior change
		Provide encouragement and "unconditional" support
		Celebrate successes
		Facebook group to provide peer social support for health behavior change
		Positive reinforcement

Ongoing support (e.g., length of interventions, text messages or calls to check in between in-person visits)	71%	Between session check-ins and avenues for support
		Intervention lasts at least 3 months
		Stepped care design (increasing/decreasing support over time and/or according to participant needs)
Shared lived experience or peer support values (e.g., experiential learning and teaching, role modeling recovery, self-disclosure, provide upward social comparison)	36%	Peers share their own experiences with health behavior change, including challenges and successes
		Engage as a co-learner to enhance peer-participation collaboration
		Role modeling
		Peer-to-peer cooperation creating a supportive network for weight loss
		Use self-disclosure to develop a non-hierarchical relationship with participants
Potential mechanisms		
Mechanism	**Percentage reporting**	**Examples**
Normalize health issues among people with mental health disorders	14%	Normalizing slips
		Being "in the same boat"
Facilitate **empowerment**	7%	
Instill **hope**	14%	
Enhance **credibility** of health-related information and advice	7%	
Promote **engagement** in health programming	21%	
Provide opportunities for **observational learning**	7%	Social influence
		Connection with and support from similar others who are making the same health behavior changes
		Group learning
Increase **self-efficacy** for health behavior change	36%	
Increase **peer support** for health behavior change	14%	
Develop **shared norms**	7%	
Increase **social relationships**	7%	Facilitate positive social interactions in a dynamic group setting

(continued)

Table 7.5 (continued)

Facilitate **non-hierarchical** relationships	7%	
Facilitate **mutual learning environment** among clinicians and peer providers	7%	
Reduce **distress**	7%	
Improve **meaningful engagement** with healthcare team	7%	
Increase **activation**	7%	
Hypothesized outcomes and documented benefits[a]		
Outcome	**Percentage reporting**	**Examples**
Improved **physical health outcomes**	86%	Weight loss[a]
		Reduction in BMI[a]
		Decreased pain[a]
Improved **health behaviors**	57%	Physical activity[a]
Increased **utilization of and engagement in routine healthcare**	21%	Scheduled and achieved appointments[a]
		Increased physical health screening[a]
		Increased visits to routine care[a]
		Health literacy[a]
		Increased detection of chronic diseases[a]
		Healthcare self-management: improved communication with provider[a]
		Improved relationship with primary care provider[a]
Reduced **acute care utilization**	7%	
Improved **quality of life or well-being**	36%	
Mental health **recovery**	36%	
Increased **healthy lifestyle goal setting**	7%	
Improved **attitudes toward physical health self-management**	7%	Self-management attitudes[a]
Housing status	7%	

Note: [a]Denotes significant findings favoring the peer support condition

approach that deserves its own mention and explanation. The Hearing Voices Network (HVN) is a network of people who hear voices, those who care for them, allies, support workers, and sympathetic mental health professionals. Ideologically grounded in the value of "expertise by experience," the HVN is guided by nine key principles, including that hearing voices is a normal human experience. A main component of this network is mutual peer support groups that offer self-help to voice hearers. The approach allows for exploration of voice experiences in a supportive and safe setting. It does not require people to identify their voices as symptoms of an illness and welcomes alternative explanations.

7.4.1.1 Contextual and Programmatic Features

Contextual and programmatic features of standalone peer support services are presented in Table 7.6. Forty-three programs were described in 32 sources. Of these, most (60%) were group interventions, 16% were delivered individually, and 21% were a hybrid of group and individual approaches. The most common intervention medium was in person (79%), followed by online (16%). About half of interventions were mutual support interventions in which supporters were not formally trained nor paid. The most common hosting organizations of these types of programs were consumer-operated service organizations (53%). Five (12%) were held at traditional behavioral healthcare organizations. Most (69%) were intended for people with SMI, while 30% were specifically for people with schizophrenia or psychosis. Of the 13 programs classified here as intended for people with schizophrenia or psychosis, nine were HVN groups intended for any people who hear voices. These groups do not require a medical diagnosis of a psychotic disorder or a biomedical understanding of the voice experience to participate. However, they were classified as intended for people with schizophrenia or psychosis as voice hearing is a common experience among people who are assigned those diagnoses and less common among the broader population of people with SMI.

7.4.1.2 Peer Support Strategies

"Being there" was the most common peer support strategy identified among standalone peer support services, with 51% of described programs explicitly mentioning a feature. This was communicated by providing avenues for socialization or participation in social leisure activities with others [61, 67, 71, 72, 78, 85, 86] and providing safe physical and emotional spaces [61–63, 65, 66, 70, 72, 78, 87]. Following "being there," social and emotional support and assistance in self-management were each identified in 35% of these programs. Somewhat surprisingly, only a third of programs specifically mentioned a strategy explicitly using shared lived experience or peer support values, such as acting as a role model or providing knowledge grounded in lived experience. Twenty-one percent of programs provided some aspect of ongoing support: four programs were not time limited (9%), one time-limited program lasted 12 months (2%), one provided between-session check-ins and support (2%), and three were available for people undergoing crises outside of

Table 7.6 Contextual and programmatic features of standalone mental health peer support interventions

Intervention characteristic	*N* (percentage)
Format	
Individual	7 (16%)
Group	26 (60%)
Hybrid	9 (21%)
Not specified	1 (2%)
Medium	
In person	34 (79%)
Online	7 (16%)
Telephone	0 (0%)
Hybrid	1 (2%)
Not specified	1 (2%)
Peer type	
Trained paid peer staff	11 (26%)
Trained volunteers	5 (12%)
Mutual support	23 (53%)
Not specified	4 (9%)
Role of peer	
Peer led	19 (44%)
Peer co-led with professional	4 (9%)
Professionally led with express encouragement of mutual support among participants	1 (2%)
Mutual support with no identified supporter	10 (23%)
Flexible	8 (19%)
Not specified	1 (2%)
Hosting organization	
Healthcare organization	0 (0%)
Behavioral healthcare organization	5 (12%)
Consumer-operated service organization	23 (53%)
Research project	2 (5%)
Other	11 (26%)
Not specified	2 (5%)
Target population	
People with SMI	29 (67%)
People with schizophrenia	13 (30%)
Not specified	1 (2%)

normal business hours (7%). Linkage to clinical care and community resources was the least represented in this category, with only 19% of programs mentioning any strategy of this type.

7.4.1.3 Potential Mechanisms

Stigma reduction was the most suggested mechanism, with 33% of programs mentioning it. Facilitating empowerment followed with 26% of programs noting this as a potential mechanism linking peer support to benefit. Also mentioned were increased social connections (21%), reduced loneliness and social isolation (19%), increased hope (16%), increased self-efficacy (7%), and increased activation (2%). As these services occurred outside of the clinical space, potential mechanisms relating to improving communication between individuals and healthcare providers or changing staff attitudes were not mentioned. However, some additional potential mechanisms emerged from the writing on these types of programs: increased insight into voices (9%), increased coping (9%), and having an emancipatory experience of reclaiming an understanding of hearing voices from a more traditional illness narrative (7%).

7.4.1.4 Hypothesized Outcomes

It is important to note that while some of the sources describing standalone peer support programs did suggest some potential benefits of their services, only one carried out a formal evaluation [88]. It may be that programs of this type are less likely to be formally studied due to their operation outside of the traditional behavioral healthcare service system. The most common hypothesized benefits of the programs were recovery outcomes (14%), followed by symptoms and functioning (9%), and care utilization (9%). Suggested benefits relating to care utilization were identified as facilitating the transition from secondary to primary care and, thereby, reducing the cost of care. Social outcomes, treatment engagement, and mental health services outcomes were also each mentioned by one program.

7.4.1.5 Significant Findings

The one standalone peer support program that was formally evaluated in a quasi-experimental study showed some significant within-group findings. Your Way, a personalized, community-based support program located in the UK, was found to significantly increase mental and physical well-being of people who received support, improve their functional living skills, and help people achieve self-directed goals [88]. The qualitative findings underscored the importance of peer support to the service users, as well as the program's approach to incremental goal setting [88].

7.4.1.6 Summary

Standalone peer support services frequently communicate "being there" for people and, in doing so, are suggested to normalize the experience of having a mental illness and reduce stigma. They have not been formally studied in most instances, so evidence of effectiveness is limited. Full details of these interventions are provided in Table 7.7.

7.4.2 Peer Support Services in Conjunction with Clinical Services

Peer support services in conjunction with clinical services were defined in this study as support that was provided in addition to, but distinct from, clinical care. This was the most common type of mental health-focused peer intervention, with 76 unique programs described in 95 sources. These include nurse-led, minimally guided mutual support groups consisting of people with psychotic disorders [89–93], a peer-delivered self-management intervention guided by a recovery workbook [94–99], peer support on inpatient units [100], and peer-delivered programs intended to support people nearing discharge from inpatient hospitalization through their transition to community living [101–106]. Furthermore, some were multicomponent interventions that included a peer support component, such as avenues for mutual support in groups facilitated by clinicians [107–110], vocational support groups as part of vocational rehabilitation services [111, 112], peer supported shared decision-making interventions [113], and digital self-monitoring interventions supported by peers [114–116].

7.4.2.1 Contextual and Programmatic Features

Descriptive statistics of the contextual and programmatic features of peer support programs provided in conjunction with clinical services are presented in Table 7.8. The most common format was group programming (42%). Eighty-two percent of programs were provided in person, 5% by telephone, and 3% online. More than half (55%) of interventions of this type employed trained paid peer staff, and 34% involved mutual support. Peers played a role in leading most interventions, independently in 39% and in conjunction with a clinical professional in 28%. Sixteen percent of these programs were clinician led with explicit encouragement of mutual support among participants and 11% involved mutual support without an identified supporter. Most were housed in a behavioral healthcare organization (64%) or a research project (21%). Slightly over half (59%) of these interventions were intended for populations of people with SMI, and the remaining 41% for people diagnosed with schizophrenia or related psychoses.

Table 7.7 Strategies, mechanisms, and outcomes of standalone peer support services ($n = 43$ programs)

Peer support strategies		
Strategy	**Percentage reporting**	**Examples**
"Being there" (e.g., socialization, companionship, conversation, validation)	51%	Socialization and leisure activities
		Safe space (validating, accepting, and allows people to listen without contributing)
		Comfortable physical space for visitors to come and do what they need to do
		Provision of spiritual sustenance
		Minimizing isolation and providing hugs
		Sense of belonging
Assistance in mental health self-management (e.g., action planning, teaching self-management skills, psychoeducation, problem-solving)	35%	Learn and practice coping skills and strategies
		Psychoeducation
		Goal setting and action planning
		Identifying and understanding triggers
		Developing wellness, prevention, or survival strategies
		Developing insight into voices
Linkage to clinical care and community resources (e.g., act as liaison between providers and patients, facilitate access to community resources, advocate for consumers with providers, promote engagement in treatment)	19%	Referral to services, including crisis hotline
		Peer advocacy
		Hospital outreach/connection with potential users while they are in inpatient care
		Signposting (providing information on other health or social care programs)
		Assistance in accessing community resources
		Service navigation (helping dealing with officialdom and bureaucracy)
Social and emotional support (e.g., provide emotional support, provide instrumental support, provide informational support)	35%	Emotional support
		Informational support
		Instrumental or practical support
		Appraisal support (encouragement and uncritical noting of inconsistencies, gaps, or areas in need of further exploration)
		Support through peer exchange and reciprocity

(continued)

Table 7.7 (continued)

Ongoing support (e.g., length of interventions, text messages or calls to check in between in-person visits)	21%	Not time-limited
		Flexible attendance permitted
		Support available outside of normal business hours for people undergoing crises
		Between session check-ins and avenues for support
		Time-limited program that lasts at least 3 months
Shared lived experience or peer support values (e.g., experiential learning and teaching, role modeling recovery, self-disclosure, provide upward social comparison)	33%	"Expertise by experience": Share relevant details of their lived experience (e.g., their perspective of what professionals say, what they found helpful)
		Mutually respectful relationships with no condescension or power imbalance
		Role modeling recovery/providing living example
		Offer alternative understanding of voice-hearing: that voices are real and meaningful and that a person's ability to cope with voices is linked to the relationship they have with them
		Lead by listening
		Promote self-determination and acknowledge that each person has a deep wisdom and expertise about managing and dealing with their own problems
		More practical, hands-on help than a professional
		Solidarity
Potential mechanisms		
Mechanism	**Percentage reporting**	**Examples**
Facilitate **empowerment**	26%	
Instill **hope**	16%	
Increase **self-efficacy** for ability to self-manage mental illness	7%	
Increased **activation**	2%	
Normalization and reduced **stigma**	33%	
Reduce **loneliness** and **social isolation**	19%	
Increase **social connections**	21%	Felt supported and cared for; listened to
		Natural community building
		Sense of belonging

"Making sense of the voices and me": Increase **insight** into voice experiences	9%	
Increase **coping**	9%	
Emancipatory experience	7%	Facilitate personalized understandings of voice hearing which can be "reclaimed" from a traditional illness narrative
		Reframing the problem
		Counteract the invalidation so often experience when people disclose experiences of psychosis
Hypothesized outcomes and documented benefits[a]		
Outcome	**Percentage reporting**	**Examples**
Care utilization	9%	Transition from secondary care to primary care
		Decreased costs
		Mental health hospital bed use
Symptoms and functioning	9%	Increased mental and physical well-being[a]
		Improvement in functional living skills[a]
Recovery outcomes	14%	Achievement of self-directed goals[a]
		Improved self-esteem
Social outcomes	2%	
Treatment engagement and adherence	2%	
Mental health **services outcomes**	2%	Increased access to interventions for mental and physical well-being

Note: [a]Denotes significant findings favoring the peer support condition

Table 7.8 Contextual and programmatic features of peer services or support in conjunction with clinical services

Intervention characteristic	*N* (percentage)
Format	
Individual	25 (33%)
Group	32 (42%)
Hybrid	15 (20%)
Not specified	4 (5%)
Medium	
In person	62 (82%)
Online	2 (3%)
Telephone	4 (5%)
Hybrid	4 (5%)
Not specified	4 (5%)
Peer type	
Trained paid peer staff	42 (55%)
Trained volunteers	5 (7%)
Mutual support	24 (32%)
Not specified	5 (7%)
Role of peer	
Peer led	30 (39%)
Peer co-led with professional	21 (28%)
Professionally led with express encouragement of mutual support among participants	12 (16%)
Mutual support with no identified supporter	8 (11%)
Flexible	1 (1%)
Not specified	4 (5%)
Hosting organization	
Healthcare organization	1 (1%)
Behavioral healthcare organization	49 (64%)
Consumer-operated service organization	4 (5%)
Research project	16 (21%)
Other	5 (7%)
Not specified	1 (1%)
Target population	
People with SMI	45 (59%)
People with schizophrenia	31 (41%)

7.4.2.2 Peer Support Strategies

Of the five key functions, assistance in mental health self-management was the most represented here, with 57% mentioning at least one strategy of this type. Following this, 43% identified linkage to clinical care or community resources and 42% "being there" or ongoing support. Relating to ongoing support, 10% of programs were not time limited [72, 107, 108, 111, 112, 117–119], and another 23% provided time-limited support lasting at least 3 months [14, 89, 90, 92, 93, 101, 120–136]. Furthermore, 4% of programs offered between session check-ins [115, 116, 121, 137], and another 4% involved a stepped care design [103, 124, 130]. Least represented here was social and emotional support. Forty-five percent of these programs identified a peer support strategy that was explicitly based on shared lived experience or another peer support value. Most reported were experiential teaching or learning (29%) [15, 94, 95, 97, 98, 100, 109, 111, 112, 124, 126, 131, 132, 135, 136, 138–150] and role modeling (24%) [14, 60, 98, 102, 103, 111, 124, 126, 135, 136, 139, 140, 143, 145, 150–153]. Two programs (3%) were completely peer developed, peer driven, and peer run [14, 154]. Finally, 9% of programs included a systems advocacy strategy.

7.4.2.3 Potential Mechanisms

Normalization of experiences leading to reduction of stigma was the most mentioned potential mechanism (30%), followed by instilling hope (25%) and increasing social connections (22%). Seventeen percent of programs endorsed each of facilitating empowerment and increasing engagement, especially among hardly reached populations. Fourteen percent suggested that reducing social isolation or loneliness was a potential mechanism linking activity to benefit, 13% noted increasing self-efficacy for mental health and daily life self-management, and 12% were viewed as supplementing a fragmented mental healthcare system. Finally, 8% noted changed attitudes among individuals and staff, 7% increased activation, and 4% each of facilitating effective communication between individuals and providers and a better understanding of individual wants and needs among mental health service providers.

7.4.2.4 Outcomes Measured

Recovery outcomes, including quality of life [93, 128, 133, 141, 144, 146, 155–157], empowerment [136, 144, 150, 158], and personal recovery [96, 103, 125, 136, 146, 157], were the most frequently measured outcomes (39%). Following this were symptoms and functioning (33%), care utilization (30%), and social outcomes (28%). Eighteen percent of programs measured mental health services outcomes, such as satisfaction with services [94–97, 130, 133, 155, 156, 159], and 17% measured treatment engagement or adherence. Five percent hypothesized change in the mental health service environment to be an outcome of peer support. Other outcomes measured included vocational and educational outcomes (3%), housing outcomes (1%), and substance use outcomes (7%).

7.4.2.5 Significant Findings

A peer support and self-management intervention delivered to individuals who had just received care from crisis response teams was described and evaluated in several publications [94–99]. In an RCT, individuals received either an intervention in which they completed a recovery workbook with the support of a peer worker or simply received the workbook in the mail. Those in the experimental group could receive up to 10 peer support sessions: 33% attended all 10 sessions and 72% attended at least three. Individuals in the peer support condition were less likely to be readmitted to acute care [94–97], remained in the community for a longer period before first readmission [94–97], and were more satisfied with the mental health services they received [94–97]. Furthermore, the intervention was found to be cost-effective at a £20,000 willingness to pay per quality-adjusted life-year [96]. There were no reported differences between the groups on recovery-related outcomes, likely because the recovery workbook was distributed to both groups. However, more people in the peer support group reported using the workbook to make written plans, perhaps increasing individuals' engagement in using the workbook to maintain stability and avoid rehospitalization [95, 97].

Another RCT of a peer support mentoring intervention designed for individuals with SMI and frequent, recurrent psychiatric hospitalizations showed significant findings favoring the peer intervention [101]. Peer recovery mentors were introduced to those they supported while still in the hospital and offered services for up to 9 months after discharge [101]. Individuals in the peer mentoring condition were less likely to be readmitted to the hospital and had longer durations of community tenure before rehospitalization [101]. They also reported greater reductions in alcohol use and psychiatric symptoms [101]. Finally, individuals in the peer mentor condition also reported greater improvement over time on physical health and hygiene [101].

An intervention consisting of family-led peer support groups that was primarily intended for caregivers and other family members of people with schizophrenia was tested in an RCT with 3 years of follow-up in China. While persons with schizophrenia were not the primary recipients of this intervention, they were encouraged to attend at least six of the most relevant group sessions and were welcome to attend all sessions. Results of the RCT indicated that those individuals with schizophrenia who were randomized to the family-led peer support intervention reported greater reductions in number and length of hospitalizations and improved functioning compared to those randomized to the control condition, which consisted of standard care and psychoeducation [121]. Furthermore, the families of the people with schizophrenia who were randomized to the family-led peer support condition also reported improved functioning compared to controls [121].

A nurse-led, minimally guided peer support group for individuals with psychotic disorders was described in several publications [89–93] and tested in an RCT [90].

In this approach, the researchers note that the presence of the nurse is crucial, offering structure, continuity, and a sense of security without actively interfering with the group process [89]. However, the nurse's role is described as facilitating peer-to-peer interaction and support. The intervention consisted of 16 group sessions of about ten participants each and was associated with decreased severity of psychopathology, including fewer negative symptoms and less distress from these symptoms compared to wait-list controls [89]. Additionally, intervention participants reported more interactions with peers outside of group sessions as well as greater increases in esteem support than controls [89, 92]. There were no significant effects of the groups on care utilization outcomes [89]. Post hoc analyses showed that those who attended more than nine sessions reported greater improvements in quality of life than those who attended less than nine sessions [92]. Additionally, costs of healthcare were lower for the high attender group than the low attender group [92].

A peer-led self-management program for people with schizophrenia implemented in Singapore consisted of six sessions combining a peer-led approach with diagnosis-specific self-management skills and was evaluated in an RCT [150]. Intervention participants reported decreased psychotic symptom severity, increased empowerment, and increased perceived recovery compared to controls [150]. One-on-one peer support over a six-month period was associated with increased self-efficacy and better quality of life compared to participants who received treatment as usual [126].

Other publications reporting quasi-experimental designs noted significant reductions in rehospitalizations [14, 107] and length of inpatient stay [118, 124] favoring the peer intervention. A peer-delivered transitional post-discharge support program was associated with significant within-group improvements in functional recovery, clinical recovery, and personal wellness [103]. Furthermore, after participating in the intervention, individuals reported being engaged in more meaningful activities [103].

Additionally, a digital app designed to increase motivation among young people with schizophrenia that included a mutual support component showed significant effects on motivated behavior, defeatist beliefs, and depression symptom severity [114]. Similarly, a small pilot study of an eight-session group intervention that combined cognitive restructuring, assertive communication skills, and peer support reported significant within-group reductions in internalized stigma and increases in satisfaction with life [138]. However, as these were multifaceted interventions that included several different components in addition to peer support, these effects cannot be causally attributed to the receipt of peer support.

7.4.2.6 Summary

Peer support services delivered in conjunction with clinical services was the most common type of peer intervention described in the literature. Considered together, interventions of this type provided the five key functions of peer support consistently, ranging from 39% of programs identifying a strategy in the social and emotional support function to 47% in assistance in mental health self-management. Forty-five percent of programs identified at least one strategy specifically grounded in shared lived experience.

Recovery outcomes, care utilization, symptoms and functioning, and social outcomes are all also measured reliably among these types of programs. Potential mechanisms linking strategy to benefit are instilling hope, reducing stigma, and increasing social connections. There is substantial evidence that peer support services delivered in conjunction with clinical care have the potential to reduce acute care utilization, improve symptoms and functioning, and promote recovery. In addition, these services can be cost-effective. Full details of these interventions are provided in Table 7.9.

7.4.3 Clinical, Paraclinical, or Case Management Services Delivered by Peers

Clinical, paraclinical, or case management services delivered by peers comprised interventions that were originally designed to be delivered by clinical, paraclinical, or case management staff and were instead delivered at least in part by peer workers. Sixteen programs of this type were described in 22 sources. Programs represented include peers as part of assertive community treatment (ACT) teams [6, 160–163]; peers delivering vocational [164–167], rehabilitation [168–173], or housing services [174]; peers facilitating the completion of psychiatric advance directives [175, 176]; and peers working as case managers [5, 7, 177, 178]. They are categorized together because the services described were initially designed or intended to be delivered by non-peer staff.

7.4.3.1 Contextual and Programmatic Features

Contextual and programmatic features of clinical, paraclinical, or case management services delivered by peers are presented in Table 7.10. Most (75%) of these programs were delivered individually and all were in-person services delivered by trained paid peer staff to people with SMI. Half were exclusively peer led, and in the other half, peers co-led with a clinical professional. Most (81%) programs took place in behavioral healthcare organizations, two (13%) as part of research projects, and one (6%) in a Center for Independent Living, a consumer-operated service organization.

7.4.3.2 Peer Support Strategies

Of the five key functions of peer support, linkage to clinical care and community resources was the most represented among these programs, with 44% of programs including a description of such. Following this, assistance in mental health self-management was described in 38% of programs and social and emotional support in 31% of programs. Interestingly, only 19% of programs were classified as providing ongoing support; however, this may be because the services described, such as

Table 7.9 Strategies, mechanisms, and outcomes of peer services or support in conjunction with clinical services ($n = 76$ programs)

Peer support strategies

Strategy	Percentage reporting	Examples
"Being there" (e.g., socialization, companionship, conversation, validation)	42%	Socialization and recreation
		Safe space to share openly
		Build warm, trusting relationships
Assistance in mental health self-management (e.g., action planning, teaching self-management skills, psychoeducation, problem-solving)	57%	Goal setting and action planning
		Teaching and sharing skills (e.g., self-management skills, coping strategies, life skills)
		Psychoeducation (topics include mental illness, stigma, healthy lifestyle, treatments, etc.)
		Relapse prevention planning
		Problem-solving
Linkage to clinical care and community resources (e.g., act as liaison between providers and patients, facilitate access to community resources, advocate for consumers with providers, promote engagement in treatment)	43%	Connect with community resources
		Connect with clinical care
		Act as an advocate and liaison between clients and clinicians
		Assist clients in developing self-advocacy skills
		Support during care transition (e.g., transition from inpatient hospitalization to community care, transitioning from FEP services to adult psychiatric services)
		Provide orientation to services
Social and emotional support (e.g., provide emotional support, provide instrumental support, provide informational support)	39%	Emotional support
		Informational support
		Instrumental or practical support
		Appraisal support
		Expanding social networks
Ongoing support (e.g., length of interventions, text messages or calls to check in between in-person visits)	42%	Not time-limited
		Between session check-ins and avenues for support
		Time-limited program that lasts at least 3 months
		Stepped care design

(continued)

Table 7.9 (continued)

Shared lived experience or peer support values (e.g., experiential learning and teaching, role modeling recovery, self-disclosure, provide upward social comparison)	45%	Role model recovery
		Experiential learning and teaching
		Peer-developed, peer-driven, peer-run
		Normalize experiences
		Mutual, non-hierarchical relationships
		Instill hope and serve as an example that recovery is possible
		Promote self-determination
		Life-oriented rather than condition focused
		Communicate empathy based on shared lived experience
		Offer genuinely alternative models of understanding
		Autonomous roles and duties (compared to paraprofessional staff)
Systems advocacy (e.g., provide staff training, challenge stigmatizing statements made by staff, provide an example of recovery to staff)	9%	Systems advocacy for recovery orientation
		Challenge stigmatizing language, attitudes, and policies
		Provide staff training
		Provide example of recovery to clinical and administrative staff
		Advocate for larger possibilities for individuals receiving care
Potential mechanisms		
Mechanism	**Percentage reporting**	**Examples**
Facilitate **empowerment**	17%	Encourage individuals to move from traditional role of client or patient to more active role involving voicing of opinions
		Empower individuals to be more outspoken about pursuing their own goals
		Increased sense of empowerment through new ways of thinking and feeling
Instill **hope**	25%	Role model for both patients and non-peer staff, encouraging both to be hopeful and action-oriented regarding recovery
		Peer support serves as a visible symbol of hope
Increase **self-efficacy** for ability to self-manage mental illness	13%	Confidence (in recovery, recognizing early warning signs, ability to self-manage, etc.)
Increased **activation**	7%	Motivation to move out of comfort zone to pursue personal goals

Normalization and reduced **stigma**	30%	Universalize issues and mitigate stigma
Reduce **loneliness** and **social isolation**	14%	Reduced sense of loneliness and feeling alone
Increase **social connections**	22%	More mutually supportive and trusting relationships
Facilitate **effective communication** between consumers and providers	4%	Facilitate self-advocacy and help individuals tell the story they want about themselves
Better **understanding** of consumer wants and needs **among mental health service providers**	4%	Improved communication and a richer understanding of individual preferences, needs, and goals
Changed **attitudes among staff and clients**	8%	Help treatment team become more patient centered
		Increased trust in providers and treatments
Facilitate **engagement** (especially among hardly reached people)	17%	Act as a bridge into services for individuals with severe mental health crises and complex treatment needs who have a distrust in mental health services
		Engage individuals in social and clinical programming
Supplement Fragmented mental health system	12%	Provision of holistic care
		Bridge the perceived gap between crisis and continuing care
		Non-judgmental approach allowed individuals the dignity of risk
		Non-directive approach allowed individuals to come to their own realizations
		Increased insight into illness experiences
Hypothesized outcomes and documented benefits[a]		
Outcome	**Percentage reporting**	**Examples**
Care utilization	30%	Rehospitalization[a]
		Length of hospital stay[a]
		Length of time to rehospitalization[a]
		Long-term hospitalization outcomes[a]
		Readmission to acute care[a]
		Time to first readmission to acute care[a]
		Cost-effectiveness[a]
		Cost of care[a]

(continued)

Table 7.9 (continued)

Symptoms and functioning	33%	Negative symptoms[a]
		Severity of psychopathology[a]
		Patient functioning[a]
		Decreased relapse[a]
		Unusual behavior[a]
		Excitement[a]
		Motivated behavior[a]
		Defeatist beliefs[a]
		Depression symptom severity[a]
		Psychotic symptom severity[a]
Recovery outcomes	39%	Internalized stigma[a]
		Satisfaction with life[a]
		Quality of life[a]
		Improved self-efficacy[a]
		Mental well-being[a]
		Recovery[a]
		Recovery is possible[a]
		Functional recovery[a]
		Clinical recovery[a]
		Personal wellness (including intellectual[a], emotional, physical, social[a], vocational, environmental, psychological[a], and spiritual)
		Engaged in more meaningful activities[a]
		Quality of life[a]
		Empowerment[a]
		Perceived recovery[a]

Social outcomes	28%	Size and content of social network[a]
		Social support[a]
		Community living skills[a]
		Family functioning[a]
		Community involvement[a]
		Social adjustment[a]
		Social functioning[a]
Vocational and educational outcomes	3%	Obtaining employment[a]
Treatment engagement and adherence	17%	Engagement in the program[a]
Mental health **services outcomes**	18%	Satisfaction with mental health services[a]
		Satisfaction with intervention[a]
Changed **mental health service environment**	5%	
Housing outcomes	1%	
Substance use	7%	Abstinence from drugs[a]
		Alcohol use[a]
Other significant outcomes		Make written recovery plans[a]
		Self-management[a]
		Physical health[a]
		Hygiene/self-care[a]
		Knowledge about illness[a]
Significant **moderator**		Morale[a]

Note: [a]Denotes significant findings favoring the peer support condition

Table 7.10 Contextual and programmatic features of clinical, paraclinical, or case management services delivered by peers

Intervention characteristic	*N* (percentage)
Format	
Individual	12 (75%)
Group	1 (6%)
Hybrid	3 (19%)
Medium	
In person	16 (100%)
Online	0 (0%)
Telephone	0 (0%)
Hybrid	0 (0%)
Peer type	
Trained paid peer staff	16 (100%)
Trained volunteers	0 (0%)
Mutual support	0 (0%)
Role of peer	
Peer led	8 (50%)
Peer co-led with professional	8 (50%)
Professionally led with express encouragement of mutual support among participants	0 (0%)
Mutual support with no identified supporter	0 (0%)
Flexible	0 (0%)
Hosting organization	
Healthcare organization	0 (0%)
Behavioral healthcare organization	13 (81%)
Consumer-operated service organization	1 (6%)
Research project	2 (13%)
Target population	
People with SMI	16 (100%)
People with schizophrenia	0 (0%)

case management, are generally not time limited and, thus, length of intervention was not thought important to mention. Finally, only one program (6%) noted any strategy that comprised "being there."

Most (69%) programs described at least one strategy that explicitly utilized an aspect of shared lived experience. This is likely because, in describing the reasoning behind employing peers to deliver these interventions, authors noted the unique capabilities and skills peers bring to the work. Most commonly, peers were described as serving as examples of recovery to both clients and staff. Finally, a quarter of programs also described how peers influenced the mental healthcare system, working to make it more patient centered and recovery oriented.

7.4.3.3 Potential Mechanisms

Half of programs noted that instilling hope was a likely mechanism connecting the provision of peer support to better outcomes. Furthermore, reflecting the clinical focus of these programs, 31% identified a better understanding of consumer needs and preferences among mental health service providers as important, 25% noted changed attitudes among staff and clients, and 25% suggested that facilitating engagement among hardly reached people was critical. Facilitating empowerment (25%) and reducing mental illness stigma (19%) were also noted in several studies. Interestingly, no sources described increased self-efficacy for self-management or the facilitation of effective communication between consumers and providers as a potential mechanism linking peer support to benefits.

7.4.3.4 Hypothesized Outcomes

Care utilization outcomes, symptoms and functioning, recovery outcomes, and mental health service outcomes were each measured by six programs (38%). Rates of acute care utilization, such as emergency department visits and inpatient hospitalizations, were hypothesized to decrease following receipt of peer-delivered services in all six studies that measured or proposed measuring these outcomes. Measured outcomes relating to symptoms and functioning included psychosis symptoms, depression, general psychiatric problems, psychological distress, crisis episodes, and functioning level. Housing and social outcomes were each measured in 19% of programs. Substance use, vocational outcomes, some aspect of treatment engagement, and the mental health service environment were each hypothesized to change because of the peer-delivered intervention in 13% of programs.

7.4.3.5 Significant Findings

Several studies in this category reported significant findings. Here, findings of equivalent outcomes between individuals who received services from peer staff compared to those who received services from non-peer staff are presented, and then, any findings that found peer-delivered services superior to professional-delivered services with respect to measured outcomes are highlighted.

In a study of consumer providers on conventional case management teams, individuals served by case management teams that included a consumer provider had comparable rates of acute care utilization, lengths of stay in acute care, use of crisis residential services, and rates of other mental health service use to those served by teams staffed entirely by non-peer staff [5, 178]. Both groups had similar rates of adherence to psychotropic medications, amount of contact with case managers, linkage to community mental health services, and retention in services [5, 178]. Post hoc analyses of retention in services found that case management teams with consumer providers were more effective at retaining clients with a diagnosis of schizophrenia or a major depressive disorder in care, and people who dropped out from these teams were more likely to be diagnosed with a personality disorder, attachment disorder, depression, or psychosis not otherwise specified. Furthermore, there were no differences between the clients served by the two different case management teams on housing stability or substance abuse [5, 178].

While the authors of this study had hypothesized that clients served by case management teams including peers would perform better on these outcomes, a finding of no difference is still remarkable, especially considering that while peer providers have considerable life experience, they tend to have less post-secondary education than mental health professionals. Furthermore, it should be noted that although the experimental group was comprised of consumer providers on conventional case management teams, there was only one consumer provider on a team of six case managers, so all participants in the experimental group did not actually receive services from the consumer provider.

Another study reported equivalent outcomes between unhoused people with SMI who received intensive case management services from consumer case managers and those who received these services from nonconsumer case managers [7]. Results showed equivalent outcomes between groups on depressive symptoms, psychotic symptoms, general psychiatric problems, quality of life, level of social support, therapeutic alliance, homelessness, and drug use [7]. These studies, both based on data from the late 1990s and early 2000s, demonstrate that employing peers as case managers is a viable staffing option, as they perform as well as non-peer staff on numerous important outcomes.

Van Vugt et al. [6] compared clients served by ACT teams that included peers with those served by ACT teams without peers and found that clients served by ACT teams that included peers had higher mental and social functioning, more met and unmet needs relating to personal recovery, and less homeless days. However, counter to the study's hypothesis, clients who were served by teams that included a peer spent more days in the hospital than those served by teams consisting of all non-peer staff [6]. The authors suggested that this relationship might be because peer providers had a heightened awareness of their clients' suffering and, thus, advocated for intervention in the form of seeking acute care [6].

Individuals who completed a psychiatric advance directive (PAD) with a peer facilitator reported statistically significant improvements on treatment satisfaction and overall empowerment, including the subscales of self-esteem and community activism [176]. Clients who completed the PAD with a non-peer facilitator had significant increases on treatment satisfaction, but not empowerment. This suggests that increasing empowerment through PAD completion may be better facilitated by a peer worker with lived experience of mental health problems than by a clinician. However, people who completed PADs in this study were satisfied with the facilitation and the completed document regardless of whether the process was facilitated by a peer or a non-peer staff.

Finally, Center for Independent Living (CIL) supports provided by peers were associated with within-group improvements over time on empowerment, recovery, quality of life, and unmet needs [169]. However, those randomized to the CIL group did not perform any differently on these outcomes than did those in the control group [169]. It should be noted that while 80% of participants randomized to the CIL group had at least one contact with a peer specialist, only slightly more than half met with their peer specialist two or more times, suggesting limited engagement with the services [169]. CIL services prioritize self-determination and, as such, do not view limited engagement in services as a flaw of the services, and peer specialists did not push engagement or suggest that it was compulsory in any way [169].

Two demonstration projects [166, 167] established that peers can provide vocational services for people with SMI, both working in conjunction with vocational specialists [166] and independently providing Individualized Placement and Support (IPS) services [167]. These demonstration projects reported a sizable percentage of their clientele getting and keeping employment; however, there was no comparison group to allow for determination of effectiveness. Similarly, Crisanti et al. [174] reported on a permanent supportive housing intervention staffed entirely by peers that was able to successfully house 61% of their clients [174]. However, there was no comparison group to allow any conclusions of the relative effectiveness of these services being provided by peers compared to non-peer professionals.

7.4.3.6 Summary

Peers delivering clinical, paraclinical, or case management services most often provided linkage to clinical care and community resources and assistance in daily self-management. Programs of this type frequently reported using strategies grounded in lived experience and noted equivalent outcomes between peer and non-peer staff on care utilization outcomes, symptoms and functioning, and mental healthcare outcomes. Programs of this type also were reported to increase recovery and improve quality of life. These outcomes were hypothesized to be achieved through the instillation of hope and the facilitation of a better understanding of individual wants and needs among care providers. Full details of these interventions are provided in Table 7.11.

7.5 Peer Intervention Focused on Improving Both Mental and Physical Health

This category included one program described in three sources. Fortuna and colleagues are currently in the process of evaluating a peer-delivered home-based medical and psychiatric self-management intervention [179–181]. This intervention aims to combine the unique perspectives of peers with the standardized delivery of evidence-based interventions through mobile health technology [179]. This research, designed through a participatory process with certified peer specialists, aims to incorporate peer philosophy into the delivery of an integrated psychiatric

Table 7.11 Strategies, mechanisms, and outcomes of clinical, paraclinical, or case management services provided by peers ($N = 16$ programs)

Peer support strategies		
Strategy	**Percentage reporting**	**Examples**
"Being there" (e.g., socialization, companionship, conversation, validation)	6%	Hold social therapeutic events as part of interactions with clients (e.g., one-on-one interactions and group activities with other clients)
Assistance in mental health self-management (e.g., action planning, teaching self-management skills, psychoeducation, problem-solving)	38%	Learn and adopt healthy coping skills
		Triage and problem-solve
		Develop recovery/resiliency/rehabilitation goals and implement plans to achieve them
		Help residents develop life skills, including interpersonal skills and living skills
Linkage to clinical care and community resources (e.g., act as liaison between providers and patients, facilitate access to community resources, advocate for consumers with providers, promote engagement in treatment)	44%	Acted as liaison between tenant and landlord for clients who obtained housing
		Ensured interagency collaboration and case management
		Facilitate completion of psychiatric advance directives (legal documents outlining preferences for one's own treatment during a future incapacitating crisis)
		Shared decision-making between providers and clients
		Informal referrals (e.g., AA, NA)
		Linkage with community-based services
		Advocate for clients
		Outreach to patients that are difficult to engage
Social and emotional support (e.g., provide emotional support, provide instrumental support, provide informational support)	31%	Provided instrumental support (e.g., worked with clients to secure housing, took clients grocery shopping)
		Provide informational support (e.g., solving problems such as transportation to work, finances)
		Facilitate support groups, including job support groups
Ongoing support (e.g., length of interventions, text messages or calls to check in between in-person visits)	19%	24/7 availability of support
		Time-limited program that lasts at least 3 months
		Stepped care design with increasing/decreasing support

Shared lived experience or peer support values (e.g., experiential learning and teaching, role modeling recovery, self-disclosure, provide upward social comparison)	69%	Disclosure of lived experience with clients
		More flexible boundaries than other members of ACT team
		Act as an example and role model of recovery (both for healthcare professionals and consumers)
		Recovery services within a group setting utilizing shared lived experiences
		"Street smarts"—knowledge grounded in lived experience
		Validate service users' experiences
		Challenge erroneous beliefs in efficacious ways because they have "been there"
		Provide care in a manner that is "less clinical" and "more positive and hopeful"
Systems advocacy (e.g., provide staff training, challenge stigmatizing statements made by staff, provide an example of recovery to staff)	25%	Provide peer expertise, patient advocacy, and consultation to the entire treatment team to promote a culture in which clients' points of view and preferences are recognized, understood, respected, and integrated into treatment
		Directly confront other members of the team and organization staff regarding discriminating comments to foster an environment of zero-tolerance
		Participate in staff training
		Inclusion of peer workers is an expression of affirmative action and consistent with civil and disability rights policies
Potential mechanisms		
Mechanism	**Percentage reporting**	**Examples**
Facilitate **empowerment**	25%	Enable self-determination
Instill **hope**	50%	Working with peers stimulated some clients to consider volunteer and/or paid work
		Optimism that they could achieve their own goals
Increased **activation**	6%	
Normalization and reduced **stigma**	19%	Reduced stigma, including self-stigma and provider stigma
Better **understanding** of consumer wants and needs **among mental health service providers**	31%	Acting as an advocate and liaison between clients and healthcare providers facilitates a better understanding of client needs
		More relevant support due to peer knowledge and insight
		Less risk of coercion in developing psychiatric advance directives

(continued)

Table 7.11 (continued)

Changed **attitudes among staff and clients**	35%	Exposure to consumer staff increased overall sensitivity and skills of non-consumer staff
		Validate service users' experiences and challenge erroneous beliefs from a "been there" viewpoint
		Facilitate greater empathy and alliance
		Changed working relationships between consumers and staff
Facilitate **engagement** (especially among hardly reached people)	25%	The ability to reach vulnerable, hardly reached populations
		Alternative pathways into treatment
		Build "natural rapport" with residents
Supplement fragmented mental health system	13%	Provision of holistic care that meets clients' needs
		Additional mode of service within the traditional treatment system
Bring about **organizational change**	6%	Implement elements of recovery-oriented care in more traditional-oriented healthcare organizations (e.g., implementation of consumer advocacy councils and participation in consumer initiative programs)
Increase general **awareness** of mental health and recovery	13%	
Positive reframing of mental illness	13%	Experience with mental illness a vocational strength not weakness
		Change attitudes about the vocational abilities of individuals who are mentally ill—those of employers and mental health professionals
Increased **social cognition**	6%	
Hypothesized outcomes and documented benefits[a,b]		
Outcome	**Percentage reporting**	**Examples**
Care utilization	38%	Acute care utilization (length of stay and number of admissions)[b]
		Mental health service utilization[b]
		Crisis episodes[b]
Symptoms and functioning	38%	Depression[b]
		Symptoms of psychosis[b]
		General psychiatric problems[b]
		Mental functioning[a]

Recovery outcomes	38%	Quality of life[b]
		Empowerment[a]
		Recovery[a]
		Quality of life
Social outcomes	19%	Level of social support[b]
		Social functioning[a]
Vocational and educational outcomes	13%	
Treatment engagement and adherence	13%	Participation in Center for Independent Living supports[a]
		Adherence to psychotropic medication[b]
		Retention in services[b]
		Amount of client contact[b]
		Linkage to needed community mental health services[a]
Mental health **services outcomes**	38%	Therapeutic alliance[b]
		Treatment satisfaction[a]
		Greater met needs[a]
		Greater unmet needs[a]
Changed **mental health service environment**	13%	Actualize recovery-oriented mental health service delivery
Housing outcomes	19%	Homelessness[b]
		Number of homeless days[a]
		Housing stability[b]
Substance use	13%	Drug use[b]
		Substance abuse[b]

Note: [a]Denotes significant findings favoring the peer support condition
[b]Denotes equivalent outcomes between peer and non-peer staff

and medical illness self-management mHealth program [179]. The resulting intervention was an adaptation of a clinician-administered self-management intervention delivered in person by peer specialists with the aid of a smartphone application [181]. Twelve different eModules were completed collaboratively with the peer specialist in weekly, one-hour, in-person sessions which the app reinforced [181]. Peers adapted their delivery of the intervention to adhere to core values of peer support, such as by encouraging self-determination by allowing individuals to select which modules they worked on each week, rather than completing them in consecutive order [179]. Furthermore, peers shared their lived experience to teach self-management skills both in-person and through text messages [179].

7.6 Refinement of Results Based on Expert Interview Feedback

Eleven participants with expertise in the field completed semi-structured interviews. Their roles relating to peer support and organizational affiliations are presented in Table 7.12.

Participants provided feedback on findings relating to contextual and programmatic features, strategies, potential mechanisms, and outcomes. A common suggestion was for a more thorough description of the nuances involved in peer support. Several interviewees referred to the continuum of peer support from formal, unidirectional peer support between employed peer workers and consumers to informal, reciprocal peer support among friends [161]. Two interviewees noted that mutual support was, in their view, a form of informal peer support, whereas programs and groups led by peer support specialists comprised formal peer support.

Among interviewees, it was contested whether programs co-led with clinicians constituted peer support, especially given that the power differential between a peer and a clinician runs the risk of silencing or severely restricting the involvement of the peer. Several respondents indicated that they didn't think programs co-led by clinicians and peers were truly peer support interventions. One respondent relayed a story of being involved in a research project that consisted of peer support groups with a psychiatrist present and felt that they were "unable to stay within [their] peer values and really see this as peer support if there is a clinician in the room, because then it becomes something other" [Participant 11]. However, another participant noted that he had been involved in research on a program co-led by a peer specialist and a psychologist and felt that it was possible to provide peer support in the presence of a clinician, if the peer role was clearly defined and was viewed as a peer support rather than "more of a case manager or a junior clinician" [Participant 4].

Relating to peer support strategies, most interview respondents underscored the fundamental value of "being there" and related many different terms for it, including "holding space" [Participant 6] and "personal connection through lived experience" [Participant 11]. Several noted that inspiring hope should be included as a peer support strategy in addition to a potential mechanism. Peers serve as an

Table 7.12 Peer support roles and organizational affiliation of interview participants

Participant ID	Peer support role(s)	Organization type
1	Mutual support group leader	Nonprofit agency—self-help
2	Chief executive officer	Nonprofit agency—advocacy
3	Mutual support group member Volunteer	Nonprofit agency—self-help
4	Researcher	University
5	Researcher	Healthcare organization
6	Mental health peer support Recovery support peer specialist Peer recovery support specialist-transition age youth Vice president	Mental health technology transfer center Peer support association
7	Mutual support group leader Director of community engagement Peer support specialist	Nonprofit agency—self-help
8	Associate vice president of peer and youth advocacy	Nonprofit agency—advocacy, education, research, and services
9	Mutual support group leader Peer support specialist	Nonprofit agency—self-help
10	Director of operations	Charitable organization—peer support
11	Chief executive officer	Charitable organization—peer support

example of what is possible and "carry the light to lead you" [Participant 7]. This is in addition to and distinct from role modeling strategies for self-management and recovery. Furthermore, an interview respondent noted that peers also role model how to get one's needs met in the service system. Finally, another stated that peers not only provide knowledge grounded in lived experience but are also able to share skills grounded in lived experience or "street smarts."

Interviewees shared varied opinions of the core or defining characteristics of peer support. Several stated that some of the key functions of peer support presented here, specifically assistance in self-management and linkage to clinical care and community resources, were only a focus of peer support if the individual themselves identified that they wanted those things. Interviewees noted that they viewed self-determination as an integral value of peer support and, as such, each person's individualized goals and preferences drove the support they received. Furthermore, one participant indicated that rather than acting as advocates for people, peers promote self-advocacy. Another participant highlighted this issue as well, noting that peers "do with" whereas clinicians tend to "do for" [Participant 11].

Finally, reduction of acute care utilization was supported by many participants as a likely outcome of many peer programs; however, nuances exist. One participant related a finding from a statewide study in Georgia [182], which showed that the introduction of peer specialists increased the amount of overall care use and

Medicaid costs, because "it helped people better navigate services" [Participant 8]. Other participants saw peer services as a different level of support that was more appropriate "when you're stable" [Participant 3]. A peer specialist stated that she did not focus on "care utilization increasing or decreasing or even just existing at all" and rather intended to "support the person in whatever they need" [Participant 6]. Further complicating the issue, one participant noted that many peer programs are focused on high-frequency users of care, which leads to findings of reduced high-cost care utilization, but "if you're focused on everyone, it might increase costs" [Participant 8]. This participant went on to recommend that policy decisions be made considering research with timelines of "more than a year, because it takes people more than a year of supports to improve... especially depending on how long [a person has] been failed by systems" [Participant 8].

References

1. Rivera JJ, Sullivan AM, Valenti SS. Adding consumer-providers to intensive case management: does it improve outcome? Psychiatr Serv. 2007;58(6):802–9.
2. Sells D, Davidson L, Jewell C, Falzer P, Rowe M. The treatment relationship in peer-based and regular case management for clients with severe mental illness. Psychiatr Serv. 2006;57(8):1179–84.
3. Clarke GN, Herinckx HA, Kinney RF, Paulson RI, Cutler DL, Lewis K, et al. Psychiatric hospitalizations, arrests, emergency room visits, and homelessness of clients with serious and persistent mental illness: findings from a randomized trial of two ACT programs vs. usual care. Ment Health Serv Res. 2000;2(3):155–64.
4. Solomon P, Draine J. One-year outcomes of a randomized trial of consumer case management. Eval Program Plann. 1995;18(2):117–27.
5. Schmidt LT, Gill KJ, Pratt CW, Solomon P. Comparison of service outcomes of case management teams with and without a consumer provider. Am J Psychiatr Rehabil. 2008;11(4):310–29. https://doi.org/10.1080/15487760802186253.
6. van Vugt MD, Kroon H, Delespaul PA, Mulder CL. Consumer-providers in assertive community treatment programs: associations with client outcomes. Psychiatr Serv. 2012;63(5):477–81. https://doi.org/10.1176/appi.ps.201000549.
7. Chinman MJ, Rosenheck R, Lam JA, Davidson L. Comparing consumer and nonconsumer provided case management services for homeless persons with serious mental illness. J Nerv Ment Dis. 2000;188(7):446–53. https://doi.org/10.1097/00005053-200007000-00009.
8. Chinman M, Oberman RS, Hanusa BH, Cohen AN, Salyers MP, Twamley EW, et al. A cluster randomized trial of adding peer specialists to intensive case management teams in the Veterans Health Administration. J Behav Health Serv Res. 2013;42(1):109–21.
9. Craig T, Doherty I, Jamieson-Craig R, Boocock A, Attafua G. The consumer-employee as a member of a Mental Health Assertive Outreach Team. I. Clinical and social outcomes. J Ment Health. 2004;13(1):59–69.
10. Sledge WH, Lawless M, Sells D, Wieland M, O'Connell MJ, Davidson L. Effectiveness of peer support in reducing readmissions of persons with multiple psychiatric hospitalizations. Psychiatr Serv. 2011;62(5):541–4.
11. O'Donnell M, Parker G, Proberts M, Matthews R, Fisher D, Johnson B, et al. A study of client-focused case management and consumer advocacy: the Community and Consumer Service Project. Aust N Z J Psychiatry. 1999;33(5):684–93.

12. Forchuk C, Martin ML, Chan Y, Jensen E. Therapeutic relationships: from psychiatric hospital to community. J Psychiatr Ment Health Nurs. 2005;12(5):556–64.
13. Letourneau N, Stewart M, Dennis CL, Hegadoren K, Duffett-Leger L, Watson B. Effect of home-based peer support on maternal–infant interactions among women with postpartum depression: a randomized, controlled trial. Int J Ment Health Nurs. 2011;20(5):345–57.
14. Chinman MJ, Weingarten R, Stayner D, Davidson L. Chronicity reconsidered: improving person-environment fit through a consumer-run service. Community Ment Health J. 2001;37(3):215–29. https://doi.org/10.1023/A:1017577029956.
15. Felton CJ, Stastny P, Shern DL, Blanch A, Donahue SA, Knight E, et al. Consumers as peer specialists on intensive case management teams: impact on client outcomes. Psychiatr Serv. 1995;46(10):1037–44. https://doi.org/10.1176/ps.46.10.1037.
16. Klein AR, Cnaan RA, Whitecraft J. Significance of peer social support with dually diagnosed clients: findings from a pilot study. Res Soc Work Pract. 1998;8(5):529–51.
17. Landers GM, Zhou M. An analysis of relationships among peer support, psychiatric hospitalization, and crisis stabilization. Community Ment Health J. 2011;47(1):106–12.
18. Min S-Y, Whitecraft J, Rothbard AB, Salzer MS. Peer support for persons with co-occurring disorders and community tenure: a survival analysis. Psychiatr Rehabil J. 2007;30(3):207.
19. Pickett SA, Diehl SM, Steigman PJ, Prater JD, Fox A, Shipley P, et al. Consumer empowerment and self-advocacy outcomes in a randomized study of peer-led education. Community Ment Health J. 2012;48(4):420–30.
20. van Gestel-Timmermans H, Brouwers EP, van Assen MA, van Nieuwenhuizen C. Effects of a peer-run course on recovery from serious mental illness: a randomized controlled trial. Psychiatr Serv. 2012;63(1):54–60.
21. Cook JA, Steigman P, Pickett S, Diehl S, Fox A, Shipley P, et al. Randomized controlled trial of peer-led recovery education using building recovery of individual dreams and goals through education and support (BRIDGES). Schizophr Res. 2012;136(1–3):36–42.
22. Cook JA, Copeland ME, Floyd CB, Jonikas JA, Hamilton MM, Razzano L, et al. A randomized controlled trial of effects of wellness recovery action planning on depression, anxiety, and recovery. Psychiatr Serv. 2012;63(6):541–7.
23. Cook JA, Copeland ME, Jonikas JA, Hamilton MM, Razzano LA, Grey DD, et al. Results of a randomized controlled trial of mental illness self-management using wellness recovery action planning. Schizophr Bull. 2011;38(4):881–91.
24. Cook JA, Copeland ME, Corey L, Buffington E, Jonikas JA, Curtis LC, et al. Developing the evidence base for peer-led services: changes among participants following wellness recovery action planning (WRAP) education in two statewide initiatives. Psychiatr Rehabil J. 2010;34(2):113–20. https://doi.org/10.2975/34.2.2010.113.120.
25. Barbic S, Krupa T, Armstrong I. A randomized controlled trial of the effectiveness of a modified recovery workbook program: preliminary findings. Psychiatr Serv. 2009;60(4):491–7.
26. Jonikas JA, Grey DD, Copeland ME, Razzano LA, Hamilton MM, Floyd CB, et al. Improving propensity for patient self-advocacy through wellness recovery action planning: results of a randomized controlled trial. Community Ment Health J. 2013;49(3):260–9.
27. Kaufmann CL, Schulberg HC, Schooler NR. Chapter 14: Self-help group participation among people with severe mental illness. Prev Hum Serv. 1995;11(2):315–31.
28. Kaplan K, Salzer MS, Solomon P, Brusilovskiy E, Cousounis P. Internet peer support for individuals with psychiatric disabilities: a randomized controlled trial. Soc Sci Med. 2011;72(1):54–62. https://doi.org/10.1016/j.socscimed.2010.09.037.
29. Proudfoot J, Parker G, Manicavasagar V, Hadzi-Pavlovic D, Whitton A, Nicholas J, et al. Effects of adjunctive peer support on perceptions of illness control and understanding in an online psychoeducation program for bipolar disorder: a randomised controlled trial. J Affect Disord. 2012;142(1–3):98–105.
30. Simon GE, Ludman EJ, Goodale LC, Dykstra DM, Stone E, Cutsogeorge D, et al. An online recovery plan program: can peer coaching increase participation? Psychiatr Serv. 2011;62(6):666–9.

31. Dennis C-L. The effect of peer support on postpartum depression: a pilot randomized controlled trial. Can J Psychiatry. 2003;48(2):115–24.
32. Dennis C-L, Hodnett E, Kenton L, Weston J, Zupancic J, Stewart DE, et al. Effect of peer support on prevention of postnatal depression among high risk women: multisite randomised controlled trial. BMJ. 2009;338:a3064.
33. Segal SP, Silverman CJ, Temkin TL. Outcomes from consumer-operated and community mental health services: a randomized controlled trial. Psychiatr Serv. 2011;62(8):915–21.
34. Davidson L, Shahar G, Stayner DA, Chinman MJ, Rakfeldt J, Tebes JK. Supported socialization for people with psychiatric disabilities: lessons from a randomized controlled trial. J Community Psychol. 2004;32(4):453–77.
35. Rogers ES, Teague GB, Lichenstein C, Campbell J, Lyass A, Chen R, et al. Effects of participation in consumer-operated service programs on both personal and organizationally mediated empowerment: results of multisite study. J Rehabil Res Dev. 2007;44:785–800.
36. Greenfield TK, Stoneking BC, Humphreys K, Sundby E, Bond J. A randomized trial of a mental health consumer-managed alternative to civil commitment for acute psychiatric crisis. Am J Community Psychol. 2008;42(1–2):135–44.
37. Bright JI, Baker KD, Neimeyer RA. Professional and paraprofessional group treatments for depression: a comparison of cognitive-behavioral and mutual support interventions. J Consult Clin Psychol. 1999;67(4):491–501. https://doi.org/10.1037//0022-006x.67.4.491.
38. Ludman EJ, Simon GE, Grothaus LC, Luce C, Markley DK, Schaefer J. A pilot study of telephone care management and structured disease self-management groups for chronic depression. Psychiatr Serv. 2007;58(8):1065–72.
39. Hunkeler EM, Meresman JF, Hargreaves WA, Fireman B, Berman WH, Kirsch AJ, et al. Efficacy of nurse telehealth care and peer support in augmenting treatment of depression in primary care. Arch Fam Med. 2000;9(8):700.
40. Sajatovic M, Howland M, Gunzler D, Kanuch SW, Cassidy KA, McCormick R, et al. Race analysis in an African American sample with serious mental illness and comorbid diabetes. Psychiatr Rehabil J. 2018;41(3):246–52. https://doi.org/10.1037/prj0000314.
41. Jerome GJ, Dalcin AT, Young DR, Stewart KJ, Crum RM, Latkin C, et al. Rationale, design and baseline data for the activating consumers to exercise through peer support (ACE trial): a randomized controlled trial to increase fitness among adults with mental illness. Ment Health Phys Act. 2012;5(2):166–74. https://doi.org/10.1016/j.mhpa.2012.05.002.
42. Muralidharan A, Niv N, Brown CH, Olmos-Ochoa TT, Fang LJ, Cohen AN, et al. Impact of online weight management with peer coaching on physical activity levels of adults with serious mental illness. Psychiatr Serv. 2018;69(10):1062–8. https://doi.org/10.1176/appi.ps.201700391.
43. Kelly EL, Braslow JT, Brekke JS. Using electronic health records to enhance a peer health navigator intervention: a randomized pilot test for individuals with serious mental illness and housing instability. Community Ment Health J. 2018;54(8):1172–9. https://doi.org/10.1007/s10597-018-0282-4.
44. Bochicchio L, Stefancic A, Gurdak K, Swarbrick M, Cabassa LJ. "We're all in this together": peer-specialist contributions to a healthy lifestyle intervention for people with serious mental illness. Admin Pol Ment Health. 2019;46(3):298–310. https://doi.org/10.1007/s10488-018-0914-6.
45. Corrigan PW, Pickett S, Schmidt A, Stellon E, Hantke E, Kraus D, et al. Peer navigators to promote engagement of homeless African Americans with serious mental illness in primary care. Psychiatry Res. 2017;255:101–3. https://doi.org/10.1016/j.psychres.2017.05.020.
46. Davenport C. Health peer support workers – agents of change bringing a lived experience workforce to support the health of people with serious mental illness. Int J Integr Care. 2018;18 https://doi.org/10.5334/ijic.s1054.
47. Illinois Institute of Technology, Access Community Health Network, Heartland Health Centers, Trilogy Behavioral Healthcare. Peer navigators to address obesity-related concerns for African Americans with serious mental illness. https://www.centerwatch.com/clinical-

trials/listings/161152/obesity-peer-navigators-address-obesity-related/&radius%3D50/ (2019). Accessed 27 May 2020.
48. Kelly E, Duan L, Cohen H, Kiger H, Pancake L, Brekke J. Integrating behavioral healthcare for individuals with serious mental illness: a randomized controlled trial of a peer health navigator intervention. Schizophr Res. 2017;182:135–41. https://doi.org/10.1016/j.schres.2016.10.031.
49. Aschbrenner KA, Naslund JA, Shevenell M, Mueser KT, Bartels SJ. Feasibility of behavioral weight loss treatment enhanced with peer support and mobile health technology for individuals with serious mental illness. Psychiatry Q. 2016;87(3):401–15. https://doi.org/10.1007/s11126-015-9395-x.
50. Johns Hopkins University, National Institute of Mental Health. Peer support for increasing physical activity in people with serious mental illnesses. https://ClinicalTrials.gov/show/NCT00458094 (2009). Accessed 12 June 2020.
51. Aschbrenner KA, Naslund JA, Shevenell M, Kinney E, Bartels SJ. A pilot study of a peer-group lifestyle intervention enhanced with mHealth technology and social media for adults with serious mental illness. J Nerv Ment Dis. 2016;204(6):483–6. https://doi.org/10.1097/NMD.0000000000000530.
52. Dartmouth-Hitchcock Medical Center, National Institute of Mental Health. Lifestyle intervention for young adults with serious mental illness. https://ClinicalTrials.gov/show/NCT02815813 (2020). Accessed.
53. University of Ottawa, Canadian Mental Health Association Ottawa Branch. Efficacy of smoking cessation treatment interventions for individuals with severe mental illness. http://www.isrctn.com/ISRCTN11353250 (2015). Accessed 26 May 2020.
54. V.A. Office of Research and Development. Peer support for exercise in older veterans with psychotic disorders. https://ClinicalTrials.gov/show/NCT02958007 (2021). Accessed 27 May 2020.
55. Young AS, Cohen AN, Goldberg R, Hellemann G, Kreyenbuhl J, Niv N, et al. Improving weight in people with serious mental illness: the effectiveness of computerized services with peer coaches. J Gen Intern Med. 2017;32(Suppl 1):48–55. https://doi.org/10.1007/s11606-016-3963-0.
56. Aschbrenner KA, Naslund JA, Gorin AA, Mueser KT, Scherer EA, Viron M, et al. Peer support and mobile health technology targeting obesity-related cardiovascular risk in young adults with serious mental illness: protocol for a randomized controlled trial. Contemp Clin Trials. 2018;74:97–106. https://doi.org/10.1016/j.cct.2018.10.005.
57. Aschbrenner KA, Naslund JA, Bartels SJ. Technology-supported peer-to-peer intervention for people with serious mental illness. Psychiatr Serv. 2016;67(8):928–9. https://doi.org/10.1176/appi.ps.670801.
58. University of California LA, Los Angeles County Department of Mental Health, University of Maryland CP. Web-based weight management for individuals with mental illness. https://ClinicalTrials.gov/show/NCT01324973 (2014). Accessed 12 June 2020.
59. Cohen AN, Young A, Goldberg R, Kreyenbuhl J, Niv N, Nowlin-Finch N, et al. Online weight management with peer supports for people with serious mental illness. Ann Behav Med. 2017;51:S691–S2.
60. Moll S, Holmes J, Geronimo J, Sherman D. Work transitions for peer support providers in traditional mental health programs: unique challenges and opportunities. Work. 2009;33(4):449–58.
61. Beavan V, de Jager A, dos Santos B. Do peer-support groups for voice-hearers work? A small scale study of hearing voices network support groups in Australia. Psychosis. 2017;9(1):57–66. https://doi.org/10.1080/17522439.2016.1216583.
62. Clarke LF. Embracing polyphoney: voices, improvisation, and the hearing voices network. Intersectionalities. 2016;5(2):1–11.

63. Dillon J, Bullimore P, Lampshire D, Chamberlin J, Read J, Dillon J. The work of experience-based experts. In: Models of madness: psychological, social and biological approaches to psychosis. 2nd ed. London: Routledge; 2013. p. 305–18.
64. Good M. Hearing Voices. Trek Magazine UBC 2015.
65. Jones N, Shattell M. Not what the textbooks describe: challenging clinical conventions about psychosis. Issues Ment Health Nurs. 2016;37(10):769–72. https://doi.org/10.1080/01612840.2016.1180725.
66. Kay G, Kendall E, Dark F. Are hearing voices networks compatible with cognitive behavioural therapy for psychosis? Aust Soc Work. 2017;70(3):312–23. https://doi.org/10.1080/0312407X.2016.1262883.
67. Oakland L, Berry K. 'Lifting the veil': a qualitative analysis of experiences in Hearing Voices Network groups. Psychosis. 2015;7(2):119–29. https://doi.org/10.1080/17522439.2014.937451.
68. Payne T, Allen J, Lavender T. Hearing Voices Network groups: experiences of eight voice hearers and the connection to group processes and recovery. Psychosis. 2017;9(3):205–15. https://doi.org/10.1080/17522439.2017.1300183.
69. Sapey B, Bullimore P. Listening to voice hearers. J Soc Work. 2013;13(6):616–32. https://doi.org/10.1177/1468017312475278.
70. Carson J. From the voices of experience, the road to recovery. Vancouver: School of Social Work and Family Studies: The University of British Columbia; 2000. p. 303.
71. Gorrindo T, Groves JE. Computer simulation and virtual reality in the diagnosis and treatment of psychiatric disorders. Acad Psychiatry. 2009;33(5):413–7. https://doi.org/10.1176/appi.ap.33.5.413.
72. NHS England. No assumptions: a narrative for personlised, coordinated care and support in mental health. Making it Real (2014).
73. Pandya A, Jan Myrick K. Wellness and recovery programs: a model of self-advocacy for people living with mental illness. J Psychiatr Pract. 2013;19(3):242–6. https://doi.org/10.1097/01.pra.0000430509.82885.d2.
74. Tan EJ, Rossell SL. Comparing how co-morbid depression affects individual domains of functioning and life satisfaction in schizophrenia. Compr Psychiatry. 2016;66:53–8. https://doi.org/10.1016/j.comppsych.2015.12.007.
75. Westreich LM. Alcohol and mental illness. Primary Psychiatry. 2005;12(1):41–64.
76. Fletcher E, Barroso A. Organizational dynamics at a peer respite: a focused ethnography of an emergent strategy. Soc Work Ment Health. 2019;17:509. https://doi.org/10.1080/15332985.2019.1579157.
77. Sweeney A, Fahmy S, Nolan F, Morant N, Fox Z, Lloyd-Evans B, et al. A mixed-methods study exploring therapeutic relationships and their association with service user satisfaction in acute psychiatric wards and crisis residential alternatives. Health Serv Delivery Res. 2014; https://doi.org/10.3310/hsdr02220.
78. Gillard S, Edwards C, Gibson S, Holley J, Owen K. New ways of working in mental health services: a qualitative, comparative case study assessing and informing the emergence of new peer worker roles in mental health services in England. Health Soc Care Delivery Res. 2014; https://doi.org/10.3310/hsdr02190.
79. Jones N, Selim AJ. Education – the rainbow at the end of the tunnel – a study of a supported education program in a consumer-operated organization, with a focus on experiences of stigma. Stockholm: Institute of Social Studies: Ersta Skondal University College; 2013. p. 50.
80. Fuller LS. The impact of peer support programs on the process of recovery from mental illness: A comparative analysis. Diss Abstr Int Sect B Sci Eng. 2010;71:2071.
81. Larsen-Barr M, Seymour F, Read J, Gibson K. Attempting to stop antipsychotic medication: success, supports, and efforts to cope. Soc Psychiatry Psychiatr Epidemiol. 2018;53(7):745–56. https://doi.org/10.1007/s00127-018-1518-x.

82. Naslund JA, Grande SW, Aschbrenner KA, Elwyn G. Naturally occurring peer support through social media: the experiences of individuals with severe mental illness using YouTube. PLoS One. 2014;9(10):e110171. https://doi.org/10.1371/journal.pone.0110171.
83. Naslund JA, Aschbrenner KA, Marsch LA, Bartels SJ. The future of mental health care: peer-to-peer support and social media. Epidemiol Psychiatr Sci. 2016;25(2):113–22. https://doi.org/10.1017/S2045796015001067.
84. Sangeorzan I, Andriopoulou P, Livanou M. Exploring the experiences of people vlogging about severe mental illness on YouTube: an interpretative phenomenological analysis. J Affect Disord. 2019;246:422–8. https://doi.org/10.1016/j.jad.2018.12.119.
85. Baumel A, Correll CU, Hauser M, Brunette M, Rotondi A, Ben-Zeev D, et al. Health technology intervention after hospitalization for schizophrenia: service utilization and user satisfaction. Psychiatr Serv. 2016;67(9):1035–8. https://doi.org/10.1176/appi.ps.201500317.
86. Schroeder R. The seriously mentally ill older adult: perceptions of the patient–provider relationship. Perspect Psychiatr Care. 2013;49(1):30–40. https://doi.org/10.1111/j.1744-6163.2012.00338.x.
87. Dillon J, Hornstein GA. Hearing voices peer support groups: a powerful alternative for people in distress. Psychosis. 2013;5(3):286–95. https://doi.org/10.1080/17522439.2013.843020.
88. Mental Health Foundation. Your way: an evaluation of a model of community mental health support developed by together for mental wellbeing. n.d.
89. Castelein S, Mulder PJ, Bruggeman R. Guided peer support groups for schizophrenia: a nursing intervention. Psychiatr Serv. 2008;59(3):326. https://doi.org/10.1176/appi.ps.59.3.326.
90. Castelein S, Bruggeman R, van Busschbach JT, van der Gaag M, Stant AD, Knegtering H, et al. The effectiveness of peer support groups in psychosis: a randomized controlled trial. Acta Psychiatr Scand. 2008;118(1):64–72. https://doi.org/10.1111/j.1600-0447.2008.01216.x.
91. Castelein S, Bruggeman R, Davidson L, van der Gaag M. Creating a supportive environment: peer support groups for psychotic disorders. Schizophr Bull. 2015;41(6):1211–3. https://doi.org/10.1093/schbul/sbv113.
92. Stant AD, Castelein S, Bruggeman R, van Busschbach JT, van der Gaag M, Knegtering H, et al. Economic aspects of peer support groups for psychosis. Community Ment Health J. 2011;47(1):99–105. https://doi.org/10.1007/s10597-009-9193-8.
93. University Medical Center Groningen. The effectiveness of support groups for people suffering from psychosis: a randomised controlled trial. http://www.isrctn.com/ISRCTN02457313 (2006).. Accessed 26 May 2020.
94. Johnson S, Mason O, Osborn D, Milton A, Henderson C, Marston L, et al. Randomised controlled trial of the clinical and cost-effectiveness of a peer-delivered self-management intervention to prevent relapse in crisis resolution team users: study protocol. BMJ Open. 2017;7(10):e015665.
95. Johnson S, Lamb D, Marston L, Osborn D, Mason O, Henderson C, et al. Peer-supported self-management for people discharged from a mental health crisis team: a randomised controlled trial. Lancet. 2018;392(10145):409–18.
96. Lloyd-Evans B, Christoforou M, Osborn D, Ambler G, Marston L, Lamb D, et al. Crisis resolution teams for people experiencing mental health crises: the CORE mixed-methods research programme including two RCTs. Progr Grants Appl Res. 2019;7(1):1–102.
97. National Institute for Health Research. Peer support may reduce readmissions following mental health crises. 2018.
98. Milton A, Lloyd-Evans B, Fullarton K, Morant N, Paterson B, Hindle D, et al. Development of a peer-supported, self-management intervention for people following mental health crisis. BMC Res Notes. 2017;10(1):588.
99. National Institute for Health Research (UK), University College London. CORE: crisis team optimisation and relapse prevention – Phase 3. http://www.isrctn.com/ISRCTN01027104 (2012). Accessed 26 May 2020.

100. Wood HJ, Brown Padilla S. Peer support work on an inpatient unit for adults experiencing psychosis. Psychosis. 2019; https://doi.org/10.1080/17522439.2019.1603321.
101. O'Connell MJ, Sledge WH, Staeheli M, Sells D, Costa M, Wieland M, et al. Outcomes of a peer mentor intervention for persons with recurrent psychiatric hospitalization. Psychiatr Serv. 2018;69(7):760–7. https://doi.org/10.1176/appi.ps.201600478.
102. Yale University, Connecticut State DoMHaAS, Eli Lilly and Company. Recovery guide intervention for recurrent psychiatric hospitalization. https://ClinicalTrials.gov/show/NCT00400166 (2009). Accessed 27 May 2020.
103. Scanlan JN, Hancock N, Honey A. Evaluation of a peer-delivered, transitional and post-discharge support program following psychiatric hospitalisation. BMC Psychiatry. 2017;17:307.
104. Kidd SA, Virdee G, Mihalakakos G, McKinney C, Feingold L, Collins A, et al. The welcome basket revisited: testing the feasibility of a brief peer support intervention to facilitate transition from hospital to community. Psychiatr Rehabil J. 2016;39(4):335–42. https://doi.org/10.1037/prj0000235.
105. Centre for Addiction and Mental Health. Testing the effectiveness of the welcome basket intervention. https://ClinicalTrials.gov/show/NCT02946255 (2019). Accessed 12 June 2020.
106. U.S. Department of Veterans Affairs, V.A. Office of Research and Development. A brief community linkage intervention for dually diagnosed individuals. https://ClinicalTrials.gov/show/NCT00137267 (2009). Accessed 12 June 2020.
107. Rice DB, Zorn A, Sigman M. The importance of structure and connection for people living with schizophrenia: a 33-year outpatient group experience. Community Ment Health J. 2018; https://doi.org/10.1007/s10597-018-0329-6.
108. Patrick V, Smith RC, Schleifer SJ, Morris ME, McLennon K. Facilitating discharge in state psychiatric institutions: a group intervention strategy. Psychiatr Rehabil J. 2006;29(3):183–8. https://doi.org/10.2975/29.2006.183.188.
109. Birchwood M, Mohan L, Meaden A, Tarrier N, Lewis S, Wykes T, et al. The COMMAND trial of cognitive therapy for harmful compliance with command hallucinations (CTCH): a qualitative study of acceptability and tolerability in the UK. BMJ Open. 2018;8(6):e021657. https://doi.org/10.1136/bmjopen-2018-021657.
110. Faith LA, Collins JO, Decker J, Grove A, Jarvis SP, Rempfer MV. Experiences of empowerment in a community cognitive enhancement therapy program: an exploratory qualitative study. Psychosis. 2019; https://doi.org/10.1080/17522439.2019.1632920.
111. Granger B, Gill P. Strategies for assisting people with psychiatric disabilities to assert their ADA rights and arrange job accommodations. Psychiatr Rehabil Skills. 2000;4(1):120–35. https://doi.org/10.1080/10973430008408399.
112. Ingraham K, Rahimi M, Tsang H, Chan F, Oulvey E. Work support groups in state vocational rehabilitation agency settings: a case study. Psychiatr Rehabil Skills. 2001;5(1):6–21. https://doi.org/10.1080/15487760108415420.
113. Goscha RJ. Finding common ground: exploring the experiences of client involvement in medication decisions using a shared decision making model. Lawrence: School of Social Welfare: University of Kansas; 2009. p. 334.
114. Schlosser DA, Campellone TR, Truong B, Etter K, Vergani S, Komaiko K, et al. Efficacy of PRIME, a mobile app intervention designed to improve motivation in young people with schizophrenia. Schizophr Bull. 2018;44(5):1010–20. https://doi.org/10.1093/schbul/sby078.
115. Allan S, Bradstreet S, Mcleod H, Farhall J, Lambrou M, Gleeson J, et al. Developing a hypothetical implementation framework of expectations for monitoring early signs of psychosis relapse using a mobile app: qualitative study. J Med Internet Res. 2019;21(10):e14366.
116. Allan S, Mcleod H, Bradstreet S, Beedie S, Moir B, Gleeson J, et al. Understanding implementation of a digital self-monitoring intervention for relapse prevention in psychosis: protocol for a mixed method process evaluation. JMIR Res Protoc. 2019;8(12):e15634.

117. Carpenter-Song E, Hipolito MMS, Whitley R. 'Right here is an oasis': how 'recovery communities' contribute to recovery for people with serious mental illnesses. Psychiatr Rehabil J. 2012;35(6):435–40. https://doi.org/10.1037/h0094576.
118. Dobson D. Rehab rounds: long-term support and social skills training for patients with schizophrenia. Psychiatr Serv. 1996;47(11):1195–6. https://doi.org/10.1176/ps.47.11.1195.
119. Waddingham R, Escher S, Dodgson G. Inner speech and narrative development in children and young people who hear voices; three perspectives on a developmental phenomenon. Psychosis. 2013;5(3):226–35. https://doi.org/10.1080/17522439.2013.845594.
120. Catalan Federation of Mental Health. Activa't per la salut mental! / "Get active!: Increase active participation of people with mental disorders and their families in their recovery processes". http://www.isrctn.com/ISRCTN15181312 (2017). Accessed 26 May 2020.
121. Chien WT, Thompson DR. An RCT with three-year follow-up of peer support groups for Chinese families of persons with schizophrenia. Psychiatr Serv. 2013;64(10):997–1005. https://doi.org/10.1176/appi.ps.201200243.
122. Chinese University of Hong Kong, Integrated Community Centers for Mental Wellness. Effect of a peer-led self-management program for recent-onset psychosis. https://ClinicalTrials.gov/show/NCT04166019 (2022). Accessed 27 May 2020.
123. Chinese University of Hong Kong, Hospital Authority HK, Jilin University Medical Science Division, Taipei Medical University. Peer-led psycho-education for schizophrenia. https://ClinicalTrials.gov/show/NCT03246932 (2020). Accessed 27 May 2020.
124. Davidson L, Stayner DA, Chinman MJ, Lambert S, Sledge WH, Martindale B, et al. Preventing relapse and readmission in psychosis: using patients' subjective experience in designing clinical interventions. In: Martindale B, editor. *Outcome studies in psychological treatments of psychotic conditions*. London: Gaskell; 2000:134–56.
125. Fundación Pública Andaluza para la Investigación de Málaga en Biomedicina y Salud, University of Alcala. Art therapy in museums in mental health recovery. https://ClinicalTrials.gov/show/NCT03985904 (2020). Accessed 12 June 2020.
126. Mahlke CI, Priebe S, Heumann K, Daubmann A, Wegscheider K, Bock T. Effectiveness of one-to-one peer support for patients with severe mental illness—a randomised controlled trial. Eur Psychiatry. 2017;42:103–10. https://doi.org/10.1016/j.eurpsy.2016.12.007.
127. Morrison A, Law H, Barrowclough C, Bentall R, Haddock G, Jones SH, et al. Psychological approaches to understanding and promoting recovery in psychosis and bipolar disorder: a mixed-methods approach. Progr Grants Appl Res. 2016;4(5):1–304.
128. National Academy of Sciences, Lentis Psychiatric Institute, GGZ Drenthe, Dimence, GGZ Friesland, GGZ Noord Holland Noord. Hospitality Project (HY): combining peer support and home-based skill training in people with schizophrenia. http://www.isrctn.com/ISRCTN14282228 (2017). Accessed 26 May 2020.
129. University of Manchester. Self-help therapy and recovery trial: evaluation of a recovery guide for psychosis. http://www.isrctn.com/ISRCTN50487713 (2010). Accessed 26 May 2020.
130. Robinson J, Bruxner A, Harrigan S, Bendall S, Killackey E, Tonin V, et al. Study protocol: the development of a pilot study employing a randomised controlled design to investigate the feasibility and effects of a peer support program following discharge from a specialist first-episode psychosis treatment Centre. BMC Psychiatry. 2010;10 https://doi.org/10.1186/1471-244X-10-37.
131. Rowe M, Bellamy C, Baranoski M, Wieland M, O'Connell MJ, Benedict P, et al. A peer-support, group intervention to reduce substance use and criminality among persons with severe mental illness. Psychiatr Serv. 2007;58(7):955–61. https://doi.org/10.1176/appi.ps.58.7.955.
132. Rowe M, Benedict P, Sells D, Dinzeo T, Garvin C, Schwab L, et al. Citizenship, community, and recovery: a group- and peer-based intervention for persons with co-occurring disorders and criminal justice histories. J Groups Addict Recover. 2009;4(4):224–44. https://doi.org/10.1080/15560350903340874.

133. University of Alberta, Alberta Health Services. Peer support experience for patients discharged from acute psychiatric care. https://ClinicalTrials.gov/show/NCT03404882 (2020). Accessed 27 May 2020.
134. The University of Hong Kong. Coaching intervention for patients with early psychosis. https://ClinicalTrials.gov/show/NCT01792856 (2015). Accessed 27 May 2020.
135. van Langen WJ, Beentjes TA, van Gaal BG, Nijhuis-van der Sanden MW, Goossens PJ. How the illness management and recovery program enhanced recovery of persons with schizophrenia and other psychotic disorders: a qualitative study. Arch Psychiatr Nurs. 2016;30(5):552–7. https://doi.org/10.1016/j.apnu.2016.04.005.
136. Livingston JD, Nijdam-Jones A, Lapsley S, Calderwood C, Brink J. Supporting recovery by improving patient engagement in a forensic mental health hospital: results from a demonstration project. J Am Psychiatr Nurses Assoc. 2013;19(3):132–45. https://doi.org/10.1177/1078390313489730.
137. Gilpin T. Service user experiences of accessing support for psychosis in rural highlands and the potential role of smartphone technology: a qualitative exploration and clinical research portfolio. Glasgow: Institue of Health and Wellbeing: University of Glasgow; 2019. p. 103.
138. Best MW, Grossman M, Milanovic M, Renaud S, Bowie CR. Be outspoken and overcome stigmatizing thoughts (boost): a group treatment for internalized stigma in first-episode psychosis. Psychosis. 2018; https://doi.org/10.1080/17522439.2018.1472630.
139. Chinman M, Lucksted A, Gresen R, Davis M, Losonczy M, Sussner B, et al. Early experiences of employing consumer-providers in the VA. Psychiatr Serv. 2008;59(11):1315–21. https://doi.org/10.1176/appi.ps.59.11.1315.
140. Kavitha M, Pfizer N. Promoting recovery through peer provided interventions – Rajah Experience. Kerala J Psychiatry. 2019;32(1):49–54.
141. McGill University Health Centre. From the darkness to being okay. Montreal: McGill University Health Centre; 2016.
142. Mental Health Foundation. Parc prison peer-led self-management project snapshot-impact report 2013–2016. Wales: Mental Health Foundation; 2016. p. 43.
143. Munson MR, Cole A, Stanhope V, Marcus SC, McKay M, Jaccard J, et al. Cornerstone program for transition-age youth with serious mental illness: study protocol for a randomized controlled trial. Trials. 2016;17(1):537. https://doi.org/10.1186/s13063-016-1654-0.
144. National Medical Research Council Singapore. Evaluation of a Peer-Led Self-Management Programme (PLSMP) for people with schizophrenia. http://www.isrctn.com/ISRCTN08387324 (2012). Accessed 26 May 2020.
145. Nicholson J, Valentine A. Key informants specify core elements of peer supports for parents with serious mental illness. Front Psychiatry. 2019;10 https://doi.org/10.3389/fpsyt.2019.00106.
146. Queen's University, St. Joseph's Healthcare Hamilton. A novel treatment approach for self-stigma in first episode psychosis. https://ClinicalTrials.gov/show/NCT03491852 (2020). Accessed 27 May 2020.
147. Rabenschlag F, Hoffmann H, Conca A, Schusterschitz C. Who benefits from peer support in psychiatric institutions? Psychiatry Q. 2012;83(2):209–20. https://doi.org/10.1007/s11126-011-9194-y.
148. Watkins S, Sanderson C, Richards V. Service user perspectives of an early intervention in psychosis service: a service evaluation. Ment Health Rev J. 2018;23(3):156–64. https://doi.org/10.1108/MHRJ-09-2017-0037.
149. West C. Powerful choices: peer support and individualized medication self-determination. Schizophr Bull. 2011;37(3):445–50. https://doi.org/10.1093/schbul/sbp053.
150. Ziqiang L. Effectiveness of the peer-led self-management Programme for people with schizophrenia in enhancing recovery: a randomized controlled trial. Singapore: Alice Lee Centre for Nursing Studies: Yong Loo Lin School of Medicine, National University of Singapore; 2017. p. 372.

151. Fan Y, Ma N, Ma L, Xu W, Lamberti JS, Caine ED. A community-based peer support service for persons with severe mental illness in China. BMC Psychiatry. 2018;18:170.
152. Rummel CB, Hansen W-P, Helbig A, Pitschel-Walz G, Kissling W. Peer-to-peer psychoeducation in schizophrenia: a new approach. J Clin Psychiatry. 2005;66(12):1580–5. https://doi.org/10.4088/JCP.v66n1214.
153. Wintrip S. From consumer to consumer-provider: a narrative analysis. London: Clinical Psychology: University of East London; 2012. p. 162.
154. Substance Abuse and Mental Health Services Administration. Peer support recovery is the future of behavioral health. Rockville: Substance Abuse and Mental Health Services Administration; 2014.
155. University Hospital Hamburg-Eppendorf. Integrated care in psychotic disorders with severe mental illness. https://www.centerwatch.com/clinical-trials/listings/162178/schizophrenia-integrated-care-psychotic-disorders/&radius%3D50/ (2018). Accessed 27 May 2020.
156. Universitätsklinikum Hamburg-Eppendorf, German Federal Ministry of Education and Research. Peer support for severe mental disorders. https://ClinicalTrials.gov/show/NCT02276469 (2014). Accessed 27 May 2020.
157. Vogel JS, Swart M, Slade M, Bruins J, van der Gaag M, Castelein S. Peer support and skills training through an eating club for people with psychotic disorders: a feasibility study. J Behav Ther Exp Psychiatry. 2019;64:80–6. https://doi.org/10.1016/j.jbtep.2019.02.007.
158. Mizock L. Development of a gender-sensitive and recovery-oriented intervention for women with serious mental illness. Psychiatr Rehabil J. 2019;42(1):3–8. https://doi.org/10.1037/prj0000313.
159. Thomas EC, Salzer MS. Associations between the peer support relationship, service satisfaction and recovery-oriented outcomes: a correlational study. J Ment Health. 2018;27(4):352–8. https://doi.org/10.1080/09638237.2017.1417554.
160. V.A. Office of Research and Development. Do consumer providers enhance recovery? https://ClinicalTrials.gov/show/NCT00781079 (2011). Accessed 27 May 2020.
161. Asad S. The role of peer support providers in inter-professional mental health care teams. Ottawa: Health Systems: Tefler School of Management, University of Ottawa; 2015.
162. Dixon L, Krauss N, Lehman A. Consumers as service providers: the promise and challenge. Community Ment Health J. 1994;30(6):615–25. https://doi.org/10.1007/BF02188599.
163. Salyers MP, Bond GR. Innovations and adaptations of assertive community treatment. Am J Psychiatr Rehabil. 2009;12(3):185–90. https://doi.org/10.1080/15487760903066289.
164. Mowbray CT, Moxley DP, Collins ME. Consumers as mental health providers: first-person accounts of benefits and limitations. J Behav Health Serv Res. 1998;25(4):397–411. https://doi.org/10.1007/BF02287510.
165. Mowbray CT, Moxley DP, Thrasher S, Bybee D, McCrohan N, Harris S, et al. Consumers as community support providers: issues created by role innovation. Community Ment Health J. 1996;32(1):47–67. https://doi.org/10.1007/bf02249367.
166. Mowbray CT, Rusilowski-Clover G, Arnold J, Allen C, Harris S, McCrohan N, et al. Project WINS: integrating vocational services on mental health case management teams. Community Ment Health J. 1994;30(4):347–62. https://doi.org/10.1007/BF02207488.
167. Kern RS, Zarate R, Glynn SM, Turner LR, Smith KM, Mitchell SS, et al. A demonstration project involving peers as providers of evidence-based, supported employment services. Psychiatr Rehabil J. 2013;36(2):99–107. https://doi.org/10.1037/h0094987.
168. Goldberg JO, Rudnick A, Roe D. Cognitive and psychiatric rehabilitation: person-centered ingredients for success. In: Serious mental illness: Person-centered approaches. London: Radcliffe Publishing; 2011. p. 271–81.
169. Salzer MS, Rogers J, Salandra N, O'Callaghan C, Fulton F, Balletta AA, et al. Effectiveness of peer-delivered Center for Independent Living supports for individuals with psychiatric disabilities: a randomized, controlled trial. Psychiatr Rehabil J. 2016;39(3):239–47. https://doi.org/10.1037/prj0000220.

170. Meurk C, Parker S, Newman E, Dark F. Staff expectations of an Australian integrated model of residential rehabilitation for people with severe and persisting mental illness: a pragmatic grounded theory analysis. Front Psych. 2019;10:468. https://doi.org/10.3389/fpsyt.2019.00468.
171. Parker S, Dark F, Newman E, Hanley D, McKinlay W, Meurk C. Consumers' understanding and expectations of a community-based recovery-oriented mental health rehabilitation unit: a pragmatic grounded theory analysis. Epidemiol Psychiatr Sci. 2019;28(4):408–17. https://doi.org/10.1017/S2045796017000749.
172. Parker S, Dark F, Newman E, Korman N, Meurk C, Siskind D, et al. Longitudinal comparative evaluation of the equivalence of an integrated peer-support and clinical staffing model for residential mental health rehabilitation: a mixed methods protocol incorporating multiple stakeholder perspectives. BMC Psychiatry. 2016;16:179.
173. Parker S, Meurk C, Newman E, Fletcher C, Swinson I, Dark F. Understanding consumers' initial expectations of community-based residential mental health rehabilitation in the context of past experiences of care: a mixed-methods pragmatic grounded theory analysis. Int J Ment Health Nurs. 2018;27(6):1650–60. https://doi.org/10.1111/inm.12461.
174. Crisanti AS, Duran D, Greene RN, Reno J, Luna-Anderson C, Altschul DB. A longitudinal analysis of peer-delivered permanent supportive housing: impact of housing on mental and overall health in an ethnically diverse population. Psychol Serv. 2017;14(2):141–53. https://doi.org/10.1037/ser0000135.
175. Tinland A, Leclerc L, Loubière S, Mougeot F, Greacen T, Pontier M, et al. Psychiatric advance directives for people living with schizophrenia, bipolar I disorders, or schizoaffective disorders: study protocol for a randomized controlled trial – daip study. BMC Psychiatry. 2019;19 https://doi.org/10.1186/s12888-019-2416-9.
176. Easter MM, Swanson JW, Robertson AG, Moser LL, Swartz MS. Impact of psychiatric advance directive facilitation on mental health consumers: empowerment, treatment attitudes and the role of peer support specialists. J Ment Health. 2020:1–9. https://doi.org/10.1080/09638237.2020.1714008.
177. Emory University, Patient-Centered Outcomes Research Institute. Engaging patients with mental disorders from the ED in outpatient care. https://ClinicalTrials.gov/show/NCT02989805 (2019). Accessed 27 May 2020.
178. Schmidt LT. Comparison of service outcomes of case management teams with and without a consumer provider. Am J Psychiatr Rehabil. 2006;66:3633.
179. Fortuna KL, Storm M, Aschbrenner KA, Bartels SJ. Integration of peer philosophy into a standardized self-management mobile health intervention. Psychiatry Q. 2018;89(4):795–800. https://doi.org/10.1007/s11126-018-9578-3.
180. Fortuna KL, Naslund JA, Aschbrenner KA, Lohman MC, Storm M, Batsis JA, et al. Text message exchanges between older adults with serious mental illness and older certified peer specialists in a smartphone-supported self-management intervention. Psychiatr Rehabil J. 2019;42(1):57–63. https://doi.org/10.1037/prj0000305.
181. Fortuna KL, Storm M, Naslund JA, Chow P, Aschbrenner KA, Lohman MC, et al. Certified peer specialists and older adults with serious mental illness' perspectives of the impact of a peer-delivered and technology-supported self-management intervention. J Nerv Ment Dis. 2018;206(11):875–81. https://doi.org/10.1097/nmd.0000000000000896.
182. Landers G, Zhou M. The impact of Medicaid peer support utilization on cost. Medicare Medicaid Res Rev. 2014;4(1):E1.

Chapter 8
Implementation Considerations and Key Challenges

A focus on implementation is necessary to close the mental health treatment gap and ensure that effective supports and services, including peer support services, reach those most in need [1]. For peer support to become embedded in routine clinical practice, key stakeholders must be willing to integrate it into existing practice and able to operationalize it effectively [2]. However, concerns about implementing peer support remain, including perceptions that it increases clinicians' workloads [3, 4]. Thus, close attention to implementation facilitators and barriers is warranted. This chapter outlines major influences on implementation identified through realist review of the literature and expands on these findings with results from key informant interviews.

8.1 Facilitators and Barriers to Successful Implementation of Peer Programs

Thirty-one of the reviewed sources included discussion of facilitators or barriers to successful implementation. In the literature, factors that facilitate successful implementation were identified, including a strong organizational recovery orientation, readiness to undertake organizational change, employment of a "critical mass" of peer supporters, and investment in organizational infrastructure to support the peer role. Implementation barriers identified include inflexible organizational adherence to a biomedical model of mental illness, unclear role descriptions, and role confusion or conflict between peer and non-peer roles. These implementation considerations are explored below.

M. Evans, *Peer Support Services Reaching People with Schizophrenia*,
https://doi.org/10.1007/978-3-031-29042-8_8

8.1.1 Organizational Culture, Recovery Orientation, and Readiness to Change

The extent to which an organization embraces a recovery philosophy was identified as important to the implementation of peer support [5–9]. A recovery-oriented mental health system prioritizes an individual's quality of life to a greater extent than symptom relief and relapse prevention [9]. While symptomatic improvement remains important in recovery-oriented care, it is not the central goal [9]. In the US, the President's New Freedom Commission on Mental Health committed in 2002 to working to transform mental health care to be more recovery oriented [10]; however, the extent to which this transformation has been realized in practice across different locations and settings is not evident. As one participant observed, "the culture and perspectives and policies in a lot of these organizations are decades behind what you would say at a conference" and went on to say "how deeply ingrained the biomedical model is in the thinking and the practices of clinical staff" [Participant 8]. Another perceived that an organization's commitment to a recovery orientation could feel performative, stating, "it's in the policy papers only as a word" [Participant 2].

Several authors noted that organizations in which the biomedical model of mental illness predominates may be pessimistic about the value of peer support and reluctant to implement it or refer people to organizations that provide it [11–13]. In writing about recovery in inpatient psychiatry, Singh and colleagues noted that settings such as inpatient wards and emergency rooms in which services tend to be very formal and structured, as well as historically grounded in a medical model, face additional challenges when trying to implement peer support programs [12]. They reported, for example, that rigid rules and protocols are frequently implemented, for ease of operating as well as safety, and this level of structure inhibits patients from making independent decisions [12]. Operating procedures such as these can be difficult to reconcile with the recovery philosophy prominent in peer support [12]. An interview participant shared his thoughts on the matter:

> I think the biggest barrier to the development of peer support in every country and it's true in [country name] because it's so biomedical, is that psychiatry as a discipline has not come to accept the recovery philosophy, you know. There are two views of recovery, there's clinical recovery which is remission held by psychiatrists, which means that you have no symptoms and return to full functionality… [name] and others, and myself, take exception to that. There can be personal recovery in which you still may have some ongoing symptoms… stabilized somewhat with medication, but that you can still live beyond limitations of mental illness, with a sense of purpose, hope, meaning, and social inclusion. Most psychiatrists don't subscribe to personal recovery; pharma certainly doesn't. [Participant 2]

Cultural change at an organizational level was identified in the realist review as a key facilitator of peer worker role adoption as well as an outcome of introducing peers into existing services, while resistance to organizational change was identified as a barrier [8]. The temporal relationship between cultural change and implementation of peer support is not necessarily straightforward. On the one hand, some authors suggested that organizations that are more recovery oriented at the outset are more likely to support implementation of peer workers [5, 7, 8, 14], but on the other hand, some also viewed hiring peer workers as a means to make an organization more recovery oriented [6, 8]. This issue was further explored in the expert interviews. While several participants agreed that peers can influence the recovery culture of organizations, they also stated that simply employing peers is not sufficient to change an organization to be recovery oriented. In the words of one participant, "that's a lot to put on a peer" [Participant 7]. In addition to employing peer workers, organizations may need to redefine their mission and goals, including creating an adequate pay structure and a career development ladder [5]. Another participant stated:

> Recovery transformation cannot be solely pursued through hiring peers. You can't expect an organization to embrace recovery just by hiring peers. It requires really an overhaul of the whole thing to become recovery oriented and peers can be one important part of that. I wouldn't rely on them to change the organization—the organization will not change, it will try to get them to change, and they'll not be really in peer roles. [Participant 4]

One participant suggested that organizations go through a readiness assessment prior to introducing peer supporters, undertake training if needed to assist in realizing recovery transformation, and then, "once the organization is ready, peers can definitely 100% make the organization much more recovery oriented" [Participant 6]. Another stated that if the organization is not ready, peer workers are "sort of left there alone… and there'll be people questioning the value of the peer support worker and patronizing him. It's much harder for [the peer worker] to do what they've been trained to do" [Participant 2]. That leadership plays a critical role in culture change was reflected by one participant, "It has to come from the top down. You can have all the motivated staff that you want, if you don't have somebody with some power championing it, it's really difficult" [Participant 10]. Studies reviewed here also found that peer workers were better integrated into services in which a good fit exists between peer support values and organizational priorities, such as quality indicators and productivity expectations [8, 15].

8.1.2 Paternalism and Peer Support: Concerns About Maintaining Recovery

The realist review identified a common concern held by non-peer staff when asked about employing peer workers—that they may not be able to handle the stresses of the job without decompensating or needing treatment [7, 12, 15, 16]. Additionally, another study noted that non-peer staff viewed peer staff as lacking sufficient knowledge of standard workplace behavior, such as calling in when sick, arriving on time, and responding in a timely manner to messages [17]. One study reported that concerns such as these could lead to the provision of flexible working practices exclusively for peer workers and a benevolent, protective approach to peers taken by the rest of the team [8]. This type of approach was noted to reinforce hierarchy within the team and preclude true integration and inclusion of peer workers as equal members of the care team [8]. Most interview participants explicitly refuted this approach, exemplified by one participant stating that "peers need things that every other employee needs" [Participant 5], including an upward mobility ladder, adequate pay, good benefits, an employee assistance program, resources to do their jobs, clear direction, and flexibility around time off.

Participants felt that reasonable accommodations for psychiatric disabilities were appropriate, but supervisors taking on the task of emotionally supporting peers is not warranted. As one participant noted, "We don't want you to police our recovery… we're fine on that. We need support in our jobs" [Participant 6]. Another participant stated that "when you're explicitly the peer support person, behaviors that would not get labeled as symptomatic for non-peers get labeled as symptomatic" [Participant 8]. Rather than focusing in on peers' vulnerabilities, the enactment of organization-wide human resources policies to support mental health and wellness among all staff was recommended.

8.1.3 "Critical Mass" of Peer Supporters

Employing a "critical mass" of peer workers was identified in the realist review as a facilitator of the successful implementation of the peer role [8, 15]. Employing at least two peer workers per community, site, or care team was purported to allow peers to adjust to their role more effectively [18] and provide peer support to each other [6]. Furthermore, Chinman and colleagues suggest that hiring a single peer places a considerable amount of stress and pressure on that individual to represent all consumers and makes it more challenging to integrate them into the workforce [6, 7]. Additionally, another study noted that having a pool of peer workers with a range of different backgrounds and experiences allowed for a better likelihood of service users finding a peer with whom they connect [8]. Finally, Chinman and colleagues [7] also noted that hiring an appropriate number of peers demonstrated to all involved that organizational leadership is committed to and values peer providers.

Interview participants also shared important insights relating to hiring enough peer supporters. While acknowledging the reality of budget limitations and differing sizes of organizations, participants recommended between two and six peer workers to be an ideal target, with higher numbers reflecting more organizational investment. For example, a research expert in the field commented, "Mostly above one. You know, two is definitely better than one, three would, I think, be better… three starts to feel like the organization is really taking it seriously" [Participant 5]. However, other participants noted that supportive infrastructure was as important or more important than sheer numbers of peers, with one stating,

> I think that [infrastructure], more than the numbers, because if you don't have that in place, it doesn't really matter what number of peer support workers you have. They're all subject

> to following a system and infrastructure that's in place, whether it's healthy or unhealthy [Participant 11].

Proper training and supervision of peer workers was noted to be a critical part of that infrastructure. Several participants recommended that supervision of peer workers be undertaken by someone who is a peer worker themselves or someone who is well trained in what the peer worker role entails, a notion that is also supported by the findings of a study included in the realist review [8]. In the words of an interview participant:

> So, at the very least there should always be another [peer worker] … I would say as well with those two, I would want a supervisor that is either a peer supporter themselves, or somebody who can go through training to get the knowledge to truly support a peer supporter as a supervisor rather than coming in from a clinical perspective and not really understanding what the role entails. [Participant 6]

Non-peer agencies contracting with peer agencies to provide supervision was suggested by several participants to achieve this, especially in organizations with a limited number of peer workers:

> I think it can work with one [peer worker] if the infrastructure is in place, and so that would have to be a contracted kind of position, with an organization that has all the pieces in place for the proper supervision and management of that particular worker in order for them not to fail. I would not leave one worker with a clinical team… that feels like a recipe for failure. But I also wouldn't leave a critical mass with a complete clinical team either… so, if you're going to invest in a critical mass, then invest in the infrastructure, invest in the proper supervision that's necessary in order to support that critical mass. [Participant 10]

However, although the preference within the field is to have peer supervisors for peer staff, one participant pointed out that, for policy reasons, this isn't always possible: "Peers aren't considered qualified mental health professionals, which some states require you to be supervised by a qualified mental health professional for billing purposes" [Participant 8].

A "community of practice" was another strategy suggested by participants to avoid tokenization of the peer role and allow peers to support each other. This involves peers supporting each other through organizations such as the Louisiana Peer Action Advocacy Coalition or the National Association of Peer Supporters. One participant stated that this type of space is not intended for discussion of specific work situations or clients, but rather dialogue about more general work-related experiences, such as encountering stigma or being asked to do tasks outside of the peer role.

8.1.4 Role Confusion and Conflict

Several studies in the realist review identified a lack of a shared understanding of the peer role, among peer and non-peer staff alike, to be a significant barrier to the successful implementation of peer workers in various settings [6, 8, 12, 17, 19–21].

Additionally, in some instances, roles were not clearly delineated and differentiated between peer and non-peer staff, creating role conflict [8, 12, 15, 20]. Participants shared their thoughts on how to avoid role conflict and confusion, emphasizing the importance of training, supervision, and regular communication and consultation between peer and non-peer leadership. Several participants suggested that in the case of non-peer organizations partnering with peer organizations to provide peer support, this could take the form of ongoing consultation between leaders from both organizations. Participants recommended preparation of organizations and non-peer staff prior to the hiring and onboarding of peers as well as the involvement of current staff in the creation of the peer role. Finally, participants endorsed certification and a peer scope of practice as helping provide clear definition to the peer role:

> Certification is still, like, somewhat controversial for some people, it depends on who, it depends on how deep in the movement you get versus the peer specialist workforce… But I think certification, right, it gives people leverage to say not only is that not in my job description, but I could lose my certification by behaving in ways that are outside of my scope and what I've been trained and certified to do… even people who don't work in peer support, part of it is just being a human in the world and at work. Like, people get pushed to do things that aren't their thing to do all the time. I think that certification can help. [Participant 8]

In a similar vein, another participant stated that measuring fidelity in research on peer support is crucial to developing a valid evidence base, as it allows for an understanding of exactly what was evaluated in the peer intervention:

> In the outcome studies, you're not 100% sure about the quality of the peer specialist services that were delivered… especially in the early days, a lot of what was happening was peers would get hired for these studies, and they were being peers for the first time, so it's not like finding established people and then having those be your interventionists. So, and because there's no fidelity measure ever used in your studies, you don't really know what you're studying. [Participant 5]

8.2 Key Issues and Challenges in the Field

In addition to implementation facilitators and barriers, there exists some major challenges within the field of peer support. Fifty-three literature sources included in the realist review discussed key challenges in the program described or in the field more generally. Below, some of the most discussed challenges are presented and expanded upon with findings from the expert interviews. Themes relating to key challenges in the field include controversies around professionalization of the peer role, negotiating boundaries, matching peer supporters with those they support, tokenism of peers, and investing in and valuing peer support. Each is discussed in turn below.

8.2.1 "Friendly Fire": Perspectives on Professionalization of the Peer Support Role

Professionalizing and credentialing the peer support workforce remains a contentious issue in the field [8, 13, 22–26]. Grounding peer support in the historical and political context of the civil rights movement from which it grew, there are concerns about peer support being co-opted by the traditional mental health system, with professionalization a large part of that co-optation [13, 24, 26]. Meurk and colleagues [15] noted that consumer-run services undergo a process of "professionalization" as a result of being integrated into the formal mental health care system and debated as to whether this professionalization is a facilitator or barrier to successful implementation.

Opinions on both sides of the issue were included in the literature reviewed. For example, Davidson and colleagues wrote that peer services in the past tended to be less formal and based on such values as flexibility, autonomy, and choice, and professionalization has caused them to be viewed by some as becoming more structured and driven by the need to attract and justify funding or reimbursement [13]. On the other hand, Gillard et al. note the advantages of formalization or professionalization include bringing respect and credibility to the role and valuing people's time and expertise by compensating them [8]. However, these authors also acknowledged that compensation, training, and titles inevitably lead to power differentials between peer workers and those they support [8]. This tension—that something that was once based in the informal or moral economy of shared experience may now be compensated by a third-party payor—was asserted to lead to feelings of alienation on the part of peer workers, especially when the promise of progressive change within the system did not materialize [23].

Interview participants acknowledged tension around this issue and further illuminated the complexity. While the participants in this study tended to endorse mostly positive aspects of professionalization of the role, they did acknowledge that there are strong opinions on both sides. One participant stated, "This is a very intense issue in the field" [Participant 8], and another acknowledged contention, saying he was "in some circles…kind of like the enemy" [Participant 5] due to his work around professionalizing the peer role in a large healthcare organization. Several participants also stated that there was ample room in the field for "a diversity of options" [Participant 4] and "multiple models" [Participant 5].

Others voiced strongly held opinions that professionalization was moving the field closer to the ideals of the recovery movement, saying that "by professionalizing peer support, we're actually kickstarting real recovery orientation within our health systems" [Participant 10] and that paying peers reflects "a shift in value system… recognizing [lived experience] as incredibly important and valid and useful and beneficial to other people who are struggling and need support" [Participant 11]. Underscoring her view of the crucial value of professionalization, one participant claimed that before the role was professional and paid, lived experience was "only undervalued, and it was nothing" [Participant 10].

Grounding these discussions in the historical context of the consumer/ex-patient/survivor movement, another participant shared her view that "in any movement, you have people who work inside systems and people who work outside systems" [Participant 8], suggesting that professionalization of peer support was an approach to transforming systems from the inside. She went on to state that while there are valid concerns on both sides of the issue, ongoing contention is not necessarily productive, saying "There's a lot of friendly fire in the peer support world and I don't think that helps" [Participant 8].

8.2.2 *Boundaries: "It's Very Fuzzy, But It's Certainly Something That We Address"*

Numerous sources reviewed here, including early work in the field as well as more recent publications, highlighted that negotiating and maintaining appropriate boundaries between peer workers and the people they support was often challenging [8, 12, 15, 25–34]. Boundaries between peers and those they support tend to be more permeable than those between clinicians and patients, especially given the value of mutuality in peer philosophy. Several authors noted that a common boundary issue encountered in peer programs was that of peers relating to those they served as friends or clients [15, 25, 26, 30, 33, 34].

Programs described in the literature differed on their approach to negotiating these boundaries. For example, one decided to enact firm professional boundaries and stressed that conversations between peers and clients should remain focused on the goal of the intervention: medication taking [28]. Another suggested that applying existing clinical boundaries to peer relationship had the potential to undermine the work and prohibit the emergence of a distinctive relationship between peers and clients as compared to relationships between clinicians and clients [8]. In a different program in which peer staff worked on teams with clinical staff, there was a concern that clients would only talk to the peer about their problems if peers did not maintain similar boundaries as clinicians [33]. The dynamic of the relationship in peer support is suggested to be more complex than that in the unidirectional provision of clinical support [8]. Timmers [26] suggested that decisions and guidelines surrounding boundaries be established prior to the development of a peer-led service.

Interview participants acknowledged that boundaries can be a "very fuzzy" issue [Participant 11], with different people and programs falling somewhere along the spectrum of professional to personal relationships. One participant indicated that the relationship was that of a "friendly acquaintance" [Participant 3], and another indicated that the rigidity of boundaries is a "personal issue" [Participant 4]. Some participants who were peer workers and mutual support group leaders stated that they were fine giving out their personal phone numbers, while others found that taking personal calls from people they support "starts to get confusing" [Participant 4]. One participant noted that there are universal ethical boundaries that peer workers must abide by, the "core things… don't date the people you support, don't sleep with the people you support, don't pay for things out of your personal money for the people you support" [Participant 8]. Additionally, this participant stated that peers do not need to be "available constantly for everybody" and "don't have to tolerate unsafe situations" [Participant 8].

Beyond those core ethical boundaries, however, another participant suggested that it "depends on how the program is structured" [Participant 6] and should be an ongoing conversation between peers and supervisors. This participant mentioned peers adding clients on social media as a boundary issue that exemplified the nuance around this issue, stating that "if it's a program for people under the age of 18, adding them on Facebook is not going to be appropriate, but if it's a program that's a clubhouse model and it's all adults, then, adding people on Facebook might be appropriate" [Participant 6]. This same participant highlighted the importance of supervisors "having an open mind and keeping whatever that peer supporter says in high regard" when considering the issue of boundaries [Participant 6].

8.2.3 "Both/And": Issues Relating to Matching Peers with Those They Support

As evidenced by the fact that two-thirds of the evidence included in the realist review was not specific to people with schizophrenia or related psychoses, diagnosis is not generally thought to be critically relevant to the experience of peer support. This sentiment was reflected among the interview participants. Some discussed ambiguities and overlap in diagnostic categories as one reason that matching by diagnosis was not advisable. Another pointed out that "it's illegal for hiring organizations to ask, 'what's your diagnosis?'" [Participant 6]. Several others noted that peer support was about so much more than the illness that matching by diagnosis was unnecessary. In the words of participants, "Peer support work is not illness specific, what you're doing is that you're addressing the common elements of what it's like to have a diagnosis of a mental illness, so the most common thing is the trauma" [Participant 2], and "If you're in crisis, anybody can probably relate who's been through a mental health challenge and who has been trained in peer support" [Participant 10]. Similarly, another participant stated:

> I don't think you have to [have] the same diagnosis. I think a big part of the peer experience is, you know, the sort of loss of agency and hope and dealing with the mental health system and not feeling heard, and I think those things are pretty universal across lots of diagnoses. So, I don't necessarily think you have to match by diagnosis. [Participant 5]

While the realist review found no empirical evidence that diagnostically matched peers are more effective or likely to engage clients, the popularity of experience-specific groups, such as Alcoholics Anonymous or the groups organized by the Hearing Voices Network, might suggest otherwise [23]. Interestingly, participants in this study who belonged, either as leaders or group members, to an illness-specific mutual support group noted that the explicit focus on schizophrenia was attractive to them, with one stating "What attracted me to [organization name] groups was that everyone pretty much had the same diagnosis, like if it wasn't schizophrenia, [it was] schizoaffective, bipolar depression with psychosis. People weren't really talking about stuff that I couldn't relate to" [Participant 3]. Another noted the group's considerations of people's unique needs that might differ by diagnosis to be important:

> Based on my own personal experience, like, I tried the [organization name] support groups, but I found that I couldn't identify with most of the people there. And so, when I found the [illness-specific organization name] support groups, there were two things. One, I could find people who could relate to what I was experiencing and two, and this was back in 2013 before everything went remote, they had a conference call, and I found that the setup was more mindful of my own needs. I have paranoia, so being in my home and making a call was easier than having to go out to a support group, where people might see me going to the group. You know, I'm of course a big proponent of being specific if you're able to. [Participant 7]

Participants also stated that while it wasn't necessary or always feasible to match by diagnosis or similar illness experience, it might be beneficial. Illustrating this, one stated:

> I think that the actual illness and the symptoms are such a small part of the peer supporter's role that it doesn't have to be the case, but I could see how, if you used to have delusions or you used to hear voices, you might have a particular affinity for people who do and could be of use to them in ways others might not be able to. So, it's a both/and I guess. [Participant 4]

Another participant noted that illness and life experiences vary widely even within diagnostic categories, and this made matching difficult:

> So, yes, it's important. Yes, people get tons of benefit, amazing benefit from having somebody with that same exact diagnosis or experience but that's going to be really rare. Even if I have depression and this other person has depression, we're going to experience it completely differently. It's, yeah, some of the symptoms are going to be the same, but they're going to have had different life influences, they're going to have different supports, they're going to have a different way of experiencing it because they're not me and so, by that token, nothing is exact. [Participant 6]

Two participants from an organization that provided peer staff to a variety of different programs noted that they generally didn't match based on diagnosis or illness experience. However, they made an exception to that general approach when it came to staffing a mobile substance withdrawal program and made it a point to seek out individuals who had substance use histories and had experienced substance withdrawal. They felt that the experience of going through substance withdrawal in community was specific enough to warrant matching based on it.

Attention to racial, ethnic, and cultural diversity, as well as other intersecting minority identities, was identified in a guidance manual included in the realist review as important for the peer support workforce [23]. Participants concurred, with one noting that shared demographics can start the peer relationship off "on more of a shared footing" [Participant 4]. Other interview participants noted the importance of cultural safety and competence regarding diversity and equity. Finally, authors highlighted other aspects of identity and experience as important, such as being a veteran [35] or a parent [27]. To be able to adequately attend to issues of identity and cultural matching, one participant underscored the importance of investing in the creation of a diverse peer workforce and letting people choose, "because you just can't tell somebody who their peer is" [Participant 8]. This participant went on to note what she felt was a broader issue in the field, that "peer has kind of become a euphemism for somebody with a psychiatric diagnosis" [Participant 8] and, because of this, the field does not fully attend to other aspects of connection and what makes a relationship truly one between peers.

8.2.4 "Everybody's Really Nice, But...": Tokenism and Peer Support

While one participant noted having seen significant improvement on this issue in the past years, most participants either related personal experiences of being tokenized as peer workers or acknowledged that tokenism was still an unfortunate reality in the field. As one put it, "it's going to be unusual that you would be with a team in which there's not going to be that" [Participant 2]. Another participant stated that a lot of times, "tokenization isn't the intent of what happened, of what people are trying to do" [Participant 6]. Participants mentioned that being the only consumer or peer representative is hard, even when they felt that their input and contributions were valued. A participant who was a peer worker and the only consumer representative on an organization's board put it succinctly, "I mean, everybody's really nice, very nice, but you know, it's, I do, I feel like I'm the token peer" [Participant 7]. Another highlighted that the combination of being the only peer and the fact that the position does not hold a lot of power both contribute to the issue:

> I think it's being the only one, and also being a little bit, you know, marginalized. So, usually, say, case management teams, they might have only one psychiatrist but because psychiatrists are a highly valued role... no one ever talks about tokenism with psychiatrists. But the combination of just being one and not having a lot of power. So, peers are typically like the lowest rung of any totem pole, usually, and so that's hard. And then that can exert pressure on peers in not beneficial ways... feeling like they're representing all peers in the eyes of their co-workers. You know, working themselves to death because they've got to maintain a certain image and it's a lot of weight, I think, to carry. [Participant 5]

One participant noted that many peer supporters often don't know they might be vulnerable to tokenization when they are offered certain opportunities:

> We've been taken advantage of for pretty much our whole lives, by the time we get to being a peer supporter and we're still trying to find out what our goal is, and then on top of that we're going into systems that don't truly understand or appreciate our role for the most part. And then they're like, "Oh, hey, we'd love for you to tell us about your experience" in this, you know, high-profile whatever. A lot of times peers are going to be like, "Yes, they're

> finally respecting me," and not understanding the detrimental impact that that could have. [Participant 6]

This participant suggested that incorporating some education around tokenism and what it looks like and how peers could respond when presented with these opportunities would be helpful. Another noted that in hiring peer workers, her organization has found that paying a few dollars above what is standard for the job in that location and investing in their peer workforce resulted in less tokenization: "Because we value individuals, we're able to attract individuals who will not be tokenized… or they call people out on it" [Participant 10].

A different participant suggested that this issue is not unique to practice and is also a major concern in research and policymaking. She relayed findings of a research study in the late 1990s that showed that, even when lived experience representation was mandated into policy decision-making, in this case after the Olmstead decision, most people with lived experience who were involved felt like their opinions weren't truly valued. She also identified that the people whose input is sought likely don't represent all perspectives: "Institutions only engage people who agree with the beliefs of dominant institutions, so the people who would disrupt, who are people with lived experience, tend to be less involved" [Participant 8].

8.2.5 "It Costs Money and Time to Actually Do Something Different": Investing in Peers

Interwoven throughout responses about a variety of other challenges in the field, participants frequently highlighted issues of low pay, limited work hours, and very few opportunities for advancement within the field. These concerns are also cited in the literature reviewed here, both historically and in recent publications [8, 24, 33, 34, 36–38]. For example, in a report of the proceedings of a policy workshop, an attendee noted that people in decision-making positions still viewed peer support as a luxury and prioritized hiring more clinicians over investing in peer support [36]. One participant who was a peer support specialist stated, "One of the biggest challenges is that we tend to not get paid as mental health professionals, when it is a profession," [Participant 6], and another noted that "most of the peer support positions are only part-time" [Participant 7]. In addition, fears about task shifting and using peers as "cheap labor" [Participants 4 & 10] were voiced by several participants. These concerns, along with few opportunities for advancement, were reported to lead to burnout and high turnover among the peer workforce:

> We want to be able to move up, we want to be able to advance in our career, and, so, if you only have peer support positions at $10 an hour, we're not going to stay with you for very long. We're going to find something else that works better and has an upward trajectory. [Participant 6]

These issues were also suggested to signal to peers that their skills and experience were not valued. In the words of one participant:

> What's most missing are opportunities for advancement. Because people want to move up in the world, they don't want to just stay doing the same job for years and years and years. If they're good at it, they'd like to be rewarded by moving up in an organization and that's difficult to do these days. They need to be valued for their lived experience, just because they were hired based on it doesn't mean that the organization necessarily values it, and people can tell when they're valued or not. [Participant 4]

Another participant noted that paying just a few dollars more than the standard for the field in their location helped them attract a "much higher quality of an applicant" [Participant 10] and stated that they then worked to communicate the value of their peers by investing in their training and certification. Furthermore, this participant noted that the organization for which she worked prioritized providing peer supervision and hiring people with lived experience of mental illness and recovery at all levels of leadership, creating opportunities for peers to advance. Participants voiced that investment in peer support and the structures and systems to support it is needed to realize its potential:

> If you don't pay people and you don't create an environment where they're financially sound and don't have to make emergency decisions about what they can do, then you're not going to be able to change culture like this, because it costs money and time to actually do something different. [Participant 8]

8.3 Looking Forward: Opportunities for Growth in the Field

Interview participants shared their thoughts on the most important things to consider about peer support for people with schizophrenia. Important areas for growth that were mentioned included expanding peer support within the first episode of psychosis programs and inpatient hospital units. Additionally, the reduction of stigma associated with schizophrenia and psychosis both within and outside mental health services was noted as a vitally important goal.

Participants saw the first episode of psychosis programs, with their focus on integrated and holistic care, as settings that could involve a range of peer support roles, including parent or family peers, mental health peers, substance use peers, and peers focused on physical health, in addition to clinical services and case management. Additionally, opportunities for young people to receive peer support was viewed as a great opportunity, with one participant stating "People shouldn't have to wait until they've been sick for 20 years to get assigned a peer. They can prevent a lot of damage from happening" [Participant 4].

Finally, the great deal of stigma experienced by people with schizophrenia or psychosis was endorsed by participants. Participants shared their own perceptions of the level of stigma associated with schizophrenia compared to other diagnostic categories, relating that it has "more trauma and more negative bias" and that "even within SMI, it's the one that gets the least respect out of anything" [Participant 3]. This stigma was reported to exist within peer support spaces as well. This was exemplified by another participant who was a peer specialist with lived experience of schizophrenia relating an interaction with another peer during training where this person made the comment, “Yeah, you and these two other people, y’all are like the most severe,” a sentiment to which she “was horrified” [Participant 7]. In the words of another participant:

> Very frankly, what I’ve seen is if you have depression, you’re not really considered SMI. And then if you have schizophrenia, you’re considered too SMI, and bipolar disorder is like this weird space where, you have a serious mental illness but, like, you don’t have schizophrenia is basically kind of how you’re treated. And, so I think that more people with, like, the experience of the diagnosis of schizophrenia or psychosis in leadership positions and explicitly talking about it is important, because it’s not fun to say that, but it’s like a secret kind of truth. [Participant 8]

Participants stated that there remains a lot of work to be done to reduce this stigma in the mental health field, including implementing person-centered policies and thoughtfully and intentionally changing the language used. Participants also suggested that employing people with these diagnoses to provide services could help to alleviate the stigma. One participant related her experience that “individuals with schizophrenia have a rich and diverse experience with their mental health challenge and make excellent peer supporters” [Participant 10]. Contrary to some people’s perceptions, it was reported that people with schizophrenia are “not just recipients of peer support, they’re peer supporters” [Participant 10].

References

1. McGinty EE, Eisenberg MD. Mental health treatment gap – the implementation problem as a research problem. JAMA Psychiatry. 2022;79(8):746–7.
2. May C. Towards a general theory of implementation. Implement Sci. 2013;8(1):1–14.
3. Gillard S, Holley J. Peer workers in mental health services: literature overview. Adv Psychiatr Treat. 2014;20(4):286–92.
4. Collins R, Firth L, Shakespeare T. “Very much evolving”: a qualitative study of the views of psychiatrists about peer support workers. J Ment Health. 2016;25(3):278–83.
5. Moll S, Holmes J, Geronimo J, Sherman D. Work transitions for peer support providers in traditional mental health programs: unique challenges and opportunities. Work. 2009;33(4):449–58.
6. Chinman M, Lucksted A, Gresen R, Davis M, Losonczy M, Sussner B, et al. Early experiences of employing consumer-providers in the VA. Psychiatr Serv. 2008;59(11):1315–21. https://doi.org/10.1176/appi.ps.59.11.1315.
7. Chinman M, Young AS, Hassell J, Davidson L. Toward the implementation of mental health consumer provider services. J Behav Health Serv Res. 2006;33(2):176–95. https://doi.org/10.1007/s11414-006-9009-3.
8. Gillard S, Edwards C, Gibson S, Holley J, Owen K. New ways of working in mental health services: a qualitative, comparative case study assessing and informing the emergence of new peer worker roles in mental health services in England. 2014. https://doi.org/10.3310/hsdr02190
9. Shepherd G, Boardman J, Slade M. Making recovery a reality. London: Sainsbury Centre for Mental Health; 2008.
10. President’s New Freedom Commission on Mental Health. Achieving the promise: transforming mental health care in America. 2003.

11. Wood HJ, Brown PS. Peer support work on an inpatient unit for adults experiencing psychosis. Psychological, Social and Integrative Approaches: Psychosis; 2019. https://doi.org/10.1080/17522439.2019.1603321.
12. Singh NN, Barber JW, Van Sant S. Handbook of recovery in inpatient psychiatry. Cham: Springer International Publishing; 2016.
13. Davidson L, Chinman M, Kloos B, Weingarten R, Stayner D, Tebes JK. Peer support among individuals with severe mental illness: a review of the evidence. Clin Psychol Sci Pract. 1999;6(2):165–87. https://doi.org/10.1093/clipsy/6.2.165.
14. Stefanovics EA, Drebing C, Sweeney P, Sofuoglu M, Rosenheck RA. Receptivity to a peer counselling program and recovery atmosphere as perceived by Veterans Health Administration peer support specialists and supervisors. Am J Psychiatr Rehabil. 2017;20(1):62–73. https://doi.org/10.1080/15487768.2016.1267050.
15. Meurk C, Parker S, Newman E, Dark F. Staff expectations of an Australian integrated model of residential rehabilitation for people with severe and persisting mental illness: a pragmatic grounded theory analysis. Front Psych. 2019;10:468. https://doi.org/10.3389/fpsyt.2019.00468.
16. Buckley P, Bahmiller D, Kenna CA, Shevitz S, Powell I, Fricks L. Resident education and perceptions of recovery in serious mental illness: observations and commentary. Acad Psychiatry. 2007;31(6):435–8. https://doi.org/10.1176/appi.ap.31.6.435.
17. Hamilton AB, Chinman M, Cohen AN, Oberman RS, Young AS. Implementation of consumer providers into mental health intensive case management teams. J Behav Health Serv Res. 2015;42(1):100–8. https://doi.org/10.1007/s11414-013-9365-8.
18. Fan Y, Ma N, Ma L, Xu W, Lamberti JS, Caine ED. A community-based peer support service for persons with severe mental illness in China. BMC Psychiatry. 2018;18:170.
19. Arbour S, Stevens A. A Recovery College in Canada: an innovative means of supporting and empowering individuals with severe mental illness. Can J Commun Ment Health. 2017;36(3):59–63. https://doi.org/10.7870/cjcmh-2017-017.
20. West C. Powerful choices: peer support and individualized medication self-determination. Schizophr Bull. 2011;37(3):445–50. https://doi.org/10.1093/schbul/sbp053.
21. Finnerty M, Austin E, Chen Q, Layman D, Kealey E, Ng-Mak D, et al. Implementation and use of a client-facing web-based shared decision-making system (mychois-commonground) in two specialty mental health clinics. Community Ment Health J. 2018;55:641. https://doi.org/10.1007/s10597-018-0341-x.
22. Styron TH, Tondora JL, Miller RA, Hunt MG, Harkness LL, Kaufman JS, et al. Community supports and inclusion. In: Yale textbook of public psychiatry. Oxford: Oxford University Press; 2016. p. 49–59.
23. Jones N. Peer involvement and leadership in early intervention in psychosis services: from planning to peer support and evaluation. 2015.
24. McCrone PR, Wright S, Zala D, Radhakrishnan Kartha M, Koeser LA, Ashworth M, et al. Location of care for people with serious mental illness (LOCAPE): implications for service use and costs using a mixed-methods approach. Health Serv Deliv Res. 2016;4:1–133.
25. Wintrip S. From consumer to consumer-provider: a narrative analysis, Clinical psychology. University of East London; 2012. p. 162.
26. Timmers T. Development of a peer counsellor program, Leadership (health). Royal Roads University; 2013. p. 168.
27. Nicholson J, Valentine A. Key informants specify core elements of peer supports for parents with serious mental illness. Front Psych. 2019;10. https://doi.org/10.3389/fpsyt.2019.00106.
28. Boardman G, Kerr D, McCann T. Peers experience of delivering a problem-solving programme to enhance antipsychotic medication adherence for individuals with schizophrenia. J Psychiatr Ment Health Nurs. 2015;22(6):423–30. https://doi.org/10.1111/jpm.12195.
29. Barrett NM, Pratt CW, Basto PM, Gill KJ. Integrating consumer providers into a service delivery system: the role of education and credentials. Psychiatr Rehabil Skills. 2000;4(1):82–104. https://doi.org/10.1080/10973430008408397.

30. Mowbray CT, Moxley DP, Collins ME. Consumers as mental health providers: first-person accounts of benefits and limitations. J Behav Health Serv Res. 1998;25(4):397–411. https://doi.org/10.1007/BF02287510.
31. Dixon L, Krauss N, Lehman A. Consumers as service providers: the promise and challenge. Community Ment Health J. 1994;30(6):615–25. https://doi.org/10.1007/BF02188599.
32. McCrone P, Wright S, Zala D, Radhakrishnan Kartha M, Koeser L, Ashworth M, et al. Location of care for people with serious mental illness (LOCAPE): implications for service use and costs using a mixed-methods approach. Health Serv Deliv Res. 2016;4:1. https://doi.org/10.3310/hsdr04340.
33. Asad S. The role of peer support providers in inter-professional mental health care teams, Health systems: Tefler School of Management. University of Ottawa; 2015.
34. Miyamoto Y, Sono T. Lessons from peer support among individuals with mental health difficulties: a review of the literature. Clin Pract Epidemiol Ment Health. 2012;8:22–9. https://doi.org/10.2174/1745017901208010022.
35. Muralidharan A, Niv N, Brown CH, Olmos-Ochoa TT, Fang LJ, Cohen AN, et al. Impact of online weight management with peer coaching on physical activity levels of adults with serious mental illness. Psychiatr Serv. 2018;69(10):1062–8. https://doi.org/10.1176/appi.ps.201700391.
36. National Academies of Sciences, Engineering, and Medicine. Key policy challenges to improve care for people with mental health and substance use disorders: proceedings of a workshop. The National Academies Press; 2020.
37. van Vugt MD, Kroon H, Delespaul PAEG, Mulder CL. Consumer-providers in assertive community treatment programs: associations with client outcomes. Psychiatr Serv. 2012;63(5):477–81. https://doi.org/10.1176/appi.ps.201000549.
38. Mowbray CT, Rusilowski-Clover G, Arnold J, Allen C, Harris S, McCrohan N, et al. Project WINS: integrating vocational services on mental health case management teams. Community Ment Health J. 1994;30(4):347–62. https://doi.org/10.1007/BF02207488.

Chapter 9
Summary, Implications, and Future Directions

9.1 Summary of Key Results

Results of the realist review organized evidence from 150 peer support programs described in the published and grey literature. Programs reviewed were classified as focusing primarily on physical health or mental health. One program focused jointly on both mental and physical health. Within programs focusing on mental health, three categories of interventions were identified: standalone peer support services, peer support services delivered in conjunction with clinical care, and clinical, paraclinical, or case management services delivered by peers. The majority were programs focused on mental health, and within those, most were peer support services delivered in conjunction with clinical services.

The categorization system utilized in this study was informed by Moll et al.'s study of work transitions among peer support providers [1]. This study found that there was a continuum of how the peer role was viewed in organizations: supplementary, complementary, or alternative to clinical services [1]. In this project, programs were classified as standalone peer support services, suggesting an alternative position; peer support in conjunction with clinical care, a complementary position; or peers delivering clinical, paraclinical, or case management services, a supplementary position. However, there are many approaches to categorizing peer interventions, and other reviews have utilized other systems. For example, Lloyd-Evans et al. [2] categorized peer interventions as mutual support groups, peer support services, and peer mental health providers, while Chinman et al. [3] classified them as peers added to traditional services, peers in existing clinical roles, and peers delivering structured curricula.

There may also be benefit in examining the contexts, strategies, mechanisms, and outcomes of peer interventions according to these or other classification systems. Positioning peer interventions on a continuum from formal to informal peer support, as suggested by Asad [4], may be particularly worthwhile to understand the

M. Evans, *Peer Support Services Reaching People with Schizophrenia*,
https://doi.org/10.1007/978-3-031-29042-8_9

nuances among these approaches. Additionally, understanding if there are important differences in strategies, mechanisms, and outcomes reported in different intervention styles (e.g., group, individual, hybrid) may provide clarity to the findings presented here, or alternately, illuminate additional areas of complexity. Future research along these lines is warranted.

9.1.1 Suggested Core Components of Peer Support for People with Schizophrenia

Analysis of the results of the realist review and key informant interviews led to the creation of an updated conceptual model. This model is intended to adequately represent the peer support strategies captured in the review and provide a framework for answering the question, "What do peer supporters do?" This framework, presented in Fig. 9.1, suggests core components of peer support interventions and provides a preliminary metric for assessing comparative effectiveness of different peer interventions. It is intended to lay out a template or typology for describing the activities undertaken in various peer support interventions and is not meant to suggest that all peer interventions must provide all core components to be considered peer support. The model depicts shared lived experience and peer support values as the basis of peer support, which influence the functions of peer support, put forth here as: (1) "being there," (2) assistance in daily self-management, (3) linkage to clinical care and community resources, (4) social and emotional support, and (5) systems advocacy. In addition, ongoing support is a key function of peer support, though not directly influenced by shared lived experience or peer support values.

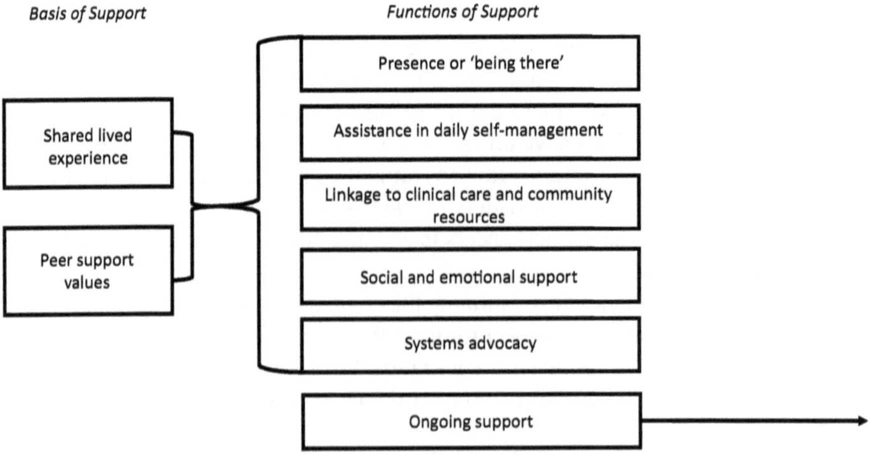

Fig. 9.1 Core components of peer support for people with schizophrenia or SMI

In the realist review, peer support activities were classified as to whether they were explicitly based on shared lived experience or peer support values. Several authors, organizations, and governing bodies have put forth lists of peer support core values [5–7]. While the wording slightly differs, common themes across these conceptualizations are that peer support is based on self-determination and autonomy as opposed to coercion, is strength focused instead of deficit focused, is characterized by a mutual relationship between equals rather than a hierarchy, and prioritizes empathy, recovery, and hope [5–7]. It is important to situate peer support as an intervention in its historical context: It began as a human and civil rights movement in which people organized around the shared experience of feeling harmed by the mental health system [8]. The core values of peer support were likely created to explicitly counter these negative experiences. These values remain today and influence the ways in which peer support is delivered that differentiate it from other types of care. For example, the core value that peer support is voluntary may determine if and how linkage to clinical care is provided, supporting the individual's choice of what services they wish to receive.

Shared lived experience also influences the way the key functions are provided. For example, peers can assist in daily self-management by sharing coping skills that were especially useful for them. Likewise, peers may have a grounded understanding of complex social service systems and how they operate due to their personal experience of navigating them, leading them to link to community resources in a different manner than clinical staff. Peers may have a deep understanding of what types of social and emotional support might be helpful to one undergoing a mental health struggle or crisis, based on having personally experienced a similar situation in the past.

Across interventions focused on physical and mental health, strategies described in the literature mapped onto the five key functions of peer support put forth by Fisher and colleagues [9–12], with some expansion of definitions. Specifically, the assistance in daily self-management function was broadened to include strategies relevant to the self-management of mental health conditions, including psychoeducation and the development of coping skills. Furthermore, this study took a liberal approach to defining linkage to clinical care and community resources. In addition to referrals to care, it included advocacy, encouragement of self-advocacy, systems navigation, and liaising between providers and patients. In addition to the original five key functions, several programs described systems advocacy as a peer support strategy. Peers acted as change agents, such as by calling out stigmatizing language, attitudes, and policies, to advance recovery-oriented care. This mostly occurred in interventions in which peers were working within clinical systems. It is important to note that these key functions could, in theory, be provided by anyone, not only a peer supporter.

The five key functions were generally endorsed by expert interviewees, and "being there" was noted as vitally important. Interview participants endorsed this concept using many different terms, including "holding space," a term for the practice of compassionately witnessing, accepting, and supporting someone without judgement, while retaining boundaries and a sense of self [13]. In designing peer support programs or training peer supporters, it is critical to uphold this fundamental value of "being there" and not minimize it in favor of the sole focus on task-oriented considerations (e.g., motivational interviewing techniques, psychoeducation). Several interviewees expressed the opinion that self-determination drives peer support activities, and in their view, assistance in self-management and linkage to clinical care and community resources generally are only undertaken as they align with the individual's goals.

Ongoing support was identified as an important aspect of peer support, although it was often overlooked in the research literature. Due to it being a function of "how" peer support is provided rather than "what" is provided, it was presented separately from the key functions in the conceptual model. Peer support consisting of the provision of the key functions is likely to be most effective when provided on an ongoing basis, as recovery can be a lifelong process. In this project, ongoing support was operationalized liberally as encompassing at least one of the following characteristics: support lasting at least 3 months, providing between-session check-ins or avenues for support, care available outside of normal business hours, or a stepped care design through which support increases or decreases according to individual needs.

In sum, from the evidence reviewed, peer support provides some combination of the following functions on an ongoing basis, informed by shared lived experience and peer support values: (1) "being there," (2) assistance in self-management, (3) linkage to clinical care or community resources, (4) social and emotional support, and (5) systems advocacy. Evaluation of the extent to which these core components were present in programs may aid in developing a better understanding how many components, which, and in what combination might be most effective.

9.1.2 Patterns of Strategies, Mechanisms, and Outcomes

The review identified peer support strategies, outcomes measured and hypothesized to change because of the intervention, and potential mechanisms linking peer support to benefit. These were then aggregated for each of the four types of programs identified: peer programs focused on physical health; standalone peer programs focused on mental health; peer support programs focused on mental health that were delivered in conjunction with clinical care; and mental health-focused clinical, paraclinical, or case management services delivered by peers. Patterns of strategies, mechanisms, and outcomes differed according to program type.

9.1.2.1 Programs Focused on Improving Physical Health

Programs focusing on improving physical health included peer group lifestyle programs to promote weight loss, peer health navigation programs, and informal peer support provided among participants of a healthy lifestyle program (e.g., via a private Facebook group). Programs of this type tended to focus heavily on assistance in self-management behaviors on an ongoing basis, with 71% of programs describing a strategy of each type. Few, however, reported a strategy that explicitly utilized shared lived experience (36%). Interestingly, a greater proportion of physical health programs reported providing ongoing support than any of the three mental health program types, in which it was described by 19–42% of programs. Research and practice implications of this finding are discussed in a subsequent section. In programs focused on physical health, the most common potential mechanisms suggested by authors included increasing self-efficacy for health behavior change (36%) and promoting engagement in health programming (21%). Important outcomes measured included improved physical health outcomes (86%) and improved health behaviors (57%).

Considering the myriad health disparities and premature mortality among this population, results that peer programs were able to achieve clinically significant weight loss [14, 15] and increased screening for and detection of chronic diseases [16, 17] are notable. These interventions were mostly for people with SMI more generally and not specifically people with schizophrenia or psychotic disorders. However, common side effects of antipsychotic medications include weight gain and increase in cardiometabolic risk, making interventions focused on physical health promotion and care navigation for people who are prescribed these medications especially important. One pilot study currently underway through the Veteran's Health Administration focuses on providing peer support to increase exercise among older veterans with psychotic disorders [18].

9.1.2.2 Mental Health-Focused Standalone Peer Support Programs

Standalone peer support programs were the least evaluated of all the program categories reviewed here. They included programs such as clubhouses, mutual support groups, alternatives to inpatient hospitalization, and informal online support. Programs of this type focused more on "being there" (51%) than the other key functions, and interestingly, only a third explicitly mentioned utilizing shared lived experience as a core component of the program. This may be thought to be self-evident; however, it was explicitly mentioned more frequently in the other program categories with a mental health focus. The most mentioned potential mechanisms were decreased stigma, increased empowerment, and increased social connections. Again, there was little focus on measuring outcomes to assess effectiveness in this category. These programs may be improved upon following formal evaluation of their effectiveness. However, these programs are likely to be conceptualized as alternatives to traditional mental health care, and those who run them may have considerable distrust in research and researchers. Peer-led research may be an ideal approach to develop evidence on this style of peer support [19].

9.1.2.3 Mental Health-Focused Peer Support Delivered in Conjunction with Clinical Care

Of the interventions focused on mental health, those provided in conjunction with clinical care were the most represented in the literature. Additionally, they tended to have the most comprehensive representation of peer support strategies, mechanisms, and outcomes. Representation of Fisher et al.'s Five Key Functions ranged from 39% of programs reporting a strategy classified as social and emotional support to 57% identifying linkage to clinical care or community resources. Almost half of programs identified the explicit utilization of shared lived experience or peer support values. In addition, 9% of programs reported that peers undertook systems advocacy. Programs of this type were most often suggested to work by reducing stigma (30%), providing hope (25%), and increasing social connections (22%). Important and frequently measured outcomes included recovery outcomes (39%), symptoms and functioning (33%), care utilization (30%), and social outcomes (28%).

9.1.2.4 Mental Health-Focused Clinical, Paraclinical, or Case Management Services Delivered by Peers

Clinical, paraclinical, or case management services delivered by peers were the least represented among the interventions focused on mental health. They included models such as ACT teams including peers and peer case managers. These interventions most often provided linkage to clinical care and community resources (44%) and assistance in self-management (38%). The most common potential mechanism suggested was instilling hope (50%). Perhaps reflecting their clinical nature, programs of this type were also hypothesized to work by facilitating a better understanding of consumer wants and needs among mental health service providers and facilitating engagement, especially among those hardly reached (25%). Care utilization (38%), symptoms and functioning (38%), recovery outcomes (38%), and changed mental health service outcomes (38%) were all commonly measured in studies of programs of this type. While studies show that peer providers of conventional case management services are as effective as non-peer providers, interview participants stressed that they did not feel that employing peers to do these jobs was necessarily a wise use of their talents. Viewing this category through the framework suggested in Fig. 9.1, the functions of peer support provided in this category may not be adequately grounded in shared lived experience or peer support values.

9.1.3 Potential Areas for Expansion

Notably absent or very infrequently measured among mental health-focused interventions were housing, vocational, and educational outcomes. These could represent areas of potential expansion for the field, especially considering the poor vocational and housing outcomes of this population. Peers who have found success in these areas may be uniquely situated to assist in ways that are practical and informed by lived experience. Many people employed as peer support specialists have navigated a return to work and could provide concrete guidance.

With their focus on integrated care and the relatively young age of the people they serve, the first episode of psychosis services seem to be an appropriate venue for providing peer support. Furthermore, providing support during the sensitive period of late adolescence and early adulthood may allow young people with psychosis to achieve their educational and vocational goals. Providing peer support early on during one's first episode of psychosis may have the potential to prevent some of the poor experiences of mental health treatment commonly reported among this population.

9.1.4 Factors Influencing the Implementation of Peer Support Programs

Facilitators and barriers to the successful implementation of peer support programs were identified in the literature and expanded upon through in-depth, semi-structured interviews with experts in the field. Issues important to consider before attempting implementation of a peer support program were identified, including the degree of organizational recovery orientation, organizational readiness to change, and capacity and willingness to invest considerable time and resources. The implementation facilitators identified here parallel those suggested as important by Glasgow et al. [23] when introducing the Chronic Care Model into health-care organizations. Barriers to the successful implementation of peer support were also identified, including role confusion and conflict, insufficient investment in peer support infrastructure, and paternalistic attitudes toward peer workers. These are also supported by current literature on the topic [20–22]. Careful attention to these factors is warranted when implementing peer support programs. Employing an implementation science framework to understand the variability in uptake and implementation of peer support services may be useful.

9.1.4.1 Recovery Transformation and the Role of Peer Support

The literature identified a shift toward a recovery orientation to be both a facilitator of the successful implementation of peer support and an outcome of introducing peer support in an organization. This finding was further explored through expert interviews in which participants stated that while peers can play a part in recovery transformation, their presence will not automatically move the organization to be more recovery oriented. Rather, interview participants asserted that trying to introduce peers into an organization that is rooted firmly in a biomedical model of mental illness and demonstrates little readiness to change may lead to peers delivering services that are not based on shared lived experience or peer support values and may be better described as paraprofessional or assistant roles than peer support.

In some ways, the focus on recovery transformation in mental health also mirrors lessons learned from the integration of the Chronic Care Model and self-management support into health-care systems to better meet the needs of patients [23]. Importantly, these authors note that teams that were most successful at integrating self-management support into their clinical workflow underwent a transformative change from viewing self-management support as an optional but nonessential component of good care to recognizing it as a central foundation of quality care [23]. Additionally, key features of the model are that it is patient centered and individualized, an iterative and self-correcting process and not a one-time activity, and an integral part of the overall health-care system design rather than a standalone, isolated activity [23]. These features of chronic illness care management might be used to further inform the process of recovery transformation in mental health services.

9.1.4.2 Key Challenges in the Field

Conflict around professionalization of the peer role, negotiating boundaries, and matching peers with those they support were highlighted in the realist review literature as key challenges in the field. A common theme identified through the interviews on the subject was that program context heavily influenced thoughts about how to best address these challenges. There were no definitive answers as to the best practices to address the following challenges, but rather a variety of good practices were suggested. Additionally, results suggest that careful consideration of the settings and contexts in which each of these good practices might be most beneficial is critical.

9.1.4.3 Professionalization

While some view professionalizing peer support as part of its co-optation by the traditional mental health system, others view it as valuing the labor of people with lived experience and a step toward true recovery transformation in systems that have been historically dominated by a biomedical paradigm. The conflicts around professionalization of the peer role, characterized by one participant as "friendly fire," demonstrate the diversity in the field regarding ideology and approach to peer support. A more productive way of approaching it might be to welcome multiple models, including paid and credentialed peer supporters as well as more informal, alternative, or disruptive approaches. This project demonstrated that there is no one best model of peer support, and diversity is a strength of the field rather than a weakness.

9.1.4.4 Negotiating Boundaries

Negotiating appropriate boundaries between peers and those they support was identified as a challenge in the field that required thoughtful consideration. Appropriate boundaries may be program specific; for example, programs involving minors being supported by adult peer workers will likely have more rigid boundaries than clubhouse models where all members are adults. Furthermore, boundaries should be developed with peer support values in mind. For example, requiring peer workers to wear staff uniforms, which may seem harmless, was identified as problematic by an interview participant. She suggested that the explicit distinction this created between peer workers and those they support negatively impacted mutuality, a core value of peer support. Findings underscored the value of attention to nuance, with no singular best practice regarding boundaries identified. Rather, standards should center ethical considerations and be thoughtfully developed for each specific program with considerable input from peer providers.

9.1.4.5 Matching

Where possible, matching peer supporters with those they support may confer a close relationship. However, it was not identified as a necessary component of establishing a peer relationship. That said, careful consideration of the situations in which matching might be especially beneficial is worthwhile. People with highly stigmatized experiences such as being diagnosed with schizophrenia might benefit from peer support from others who can relate. The existence of disorder- or experience-specific support groups and the value found in them by interview participants in this project suggests that tailoring in this manner can be a valued method to address concerns specific to schizophrenia or related disorders. However, it was also suggested by the evidence reviewed here as well as by interview participants that there are numerous other aspects of the experience of being diagnosed with and experiencing mental illness that are also important, such as the shared experience of trauma. Again, this suggests the value of multiple models of peer programs.

9.2 Study Strengths

This study had several strengths. First, the realist review methodology proved to be an innovative approach to literature review and allowed for the recognition of peer support as a complex intervention, with its success heavily dependent upon context and implementation. Second, utilizing inclusive search terms and inclusion criteria yielded a sample of diverse evidence sources from several countries, including some from low- and middle-income countries such as China and India. This is a strength as much of the peer support literature originates from high-income countries in the West. The realist review methodology and the large sample of included sources from both the published and grey literature allowed for a nuanced examination of the contexts, strategies, mechanisms, and outcomes of a variety of different types of peer interventions. Furthermore, the results from the realist review were presented to key stakeholders in the field and refined with their input, a methodological requirement in realist review [24]. Through this step, areas for theory refinement were identified, and recommendations for implementation were clarified. Together, these research activities combined the strengths of systematic literature review with an attentiveness to practical considerations which facilitated comprehensiveness in the presentation of results from a diverse and growing field.

9.3 Study Limitations

There are also several limitations of this study that should be noted. First, the realist approach to evidence synthesis does not allow us to make inferences about causality in a successionist, or experimental, paradigm. Second, the liberal inclusion criteria, while allowing for a nuanced understanding of the complexity of the field, may have complicated the realist review methodology and precluded drawing simple conclusions. Each category of peer intervention could potentially have been the subject of its own review. While considerable data reduction techniques were utilized, such as grouping like intervention strategies and mechanisms together, there may still exist some overlap in definitions of constructs presented here as distinct. For example, self-efficacy, empowerment, and patient activation are related and could potentially have been grouped together under one potential mechanism, even as definitions vary slightly among them. The degree of specificity may be adjusted in future iterations of this work.

Additionally, the sample of expert interviews may not be representative of the field as a whole. For example, interview participants tended to fall on the side of "pro-professionalization" of the peer role, and it is possible that the sampling strategy favored those who were representatives of well-known organizations with peer support programs. The sample perhaps did not adequately represent the "peer-developed peer support" faction of the broader peer support field [19]. Finally, the diversity in roles of interview participants provided a broad view of the field, while a more focused sample may have provided more depth.

9.4 Implications for Research and Practice

This study raised several important considerations for research and practice, discussed below.

9.4.1 *Evaluating Effectiveness of the Core Components of Peer Support*

The proposed core components of peer support presented here may be utilized as a framework for assessing effectiveness of peer interventions. The realist review made explicit that a wide range of activities fall under the umbrella term "peer support," and as such, assessing their effectiveness as a category may be futile. Rather, an approach of testing core components of support on specific outcomes may advance practice by informing the intentional design of peer support services to be the most effective in their desired purpose. Undertaking a qualitative comparative analysis as a next step to this research would allow for the analysis of causal complexity [25]. For example, using the core components of peer support set out in this research, a qualitative comparative analysis could illuminate the combinations of components that are successful in reducing acute care utilization among people with SMI. Alternatively, an analysis that determines the number of core components associated with effectiveness would also be informative. Analyses such as these could inform the design of programs intended to achieve these outcomes so that they are designed and delivered in ways that are more likely to have desired outcomes.

9.4.2 *Intervention Dose and Ongoing Support*

The finding that a higher proportion of peer interventions focused on physical health provided ongoing support than those focused on mental health deserves attention. It raises the question of the length of peer support, or intervention dose, needed to achieve significant mental health benefits. The need for ongoing support in physical health self-management and health behavior change is widely acknowledged in chronic disease care. For example, the American Diabetes Association, the American Association of Diabetes Educators, and the Academy of Nutrition and Dietetics all recognize that diabetes self-management support is needed on an ongoing basis to help people with diabetes implement and sustain coping skills and self-management behaviors [26].

Mental health self-management, like physical health self-management, is an ongoing process and likely requires significant investment of time to achieve clinically and personally relevant outcomes. However, there appears to be insufficient attention to providing ongoing support in peer interventions to improve mental health and promote recovery. This was evidenced here by the low proportion of mental health-focused peer programs lasting at least 3 months, ranging from 11% for standalone peer support services and clinical, paraclinical, or case management services delivered by peers to 33% for peer support in conjunction with clinical care. Learning to live with and effectively manage a condition such as schizophrenia is likely just as challenging, if not more so, than learning to live with and effectively manage diabetes. As such, ongoing support should be a critical aspect to consider when conceptualizing, delivering, and evaluating mental health peer support programs. Research on peer support may also benefit from longer intervention and follow-up observation periods.

Several recent publications reporting null findings of peer support can also be examined considering intervention dose. For example, an RCT of a peer-led transitional discharge intervention consisted of five contacts in the full-scale intervention and was abbreviated to only two contacts in a brief version [27]. The original conceptualization of this intervention involved several months of follow-up and was found to be effective in reducing acute care utilization [28, 29]. Another recent large-scale RCT of a peer intervention intended to reduce rehospitalization found no benefit. However, the intervention was characterized by poor engagement, achieving an average of only 6 of 14 planned contacts over a period of 4 months [30]. Furthermore, rehospitalization was less likely among participants who received at least two peer support sessions compared to controls, showing a dose-response relationship [30]. While these trials do address a documented limitation in the evidence base, a dearth of high-quality clinical trials, the authors' conceptualization of peer support as a relatively brief intervention as well as poor engagement preclude drawing definitive conclusions about the effectiveness of ongoing peer support on acute care utilization outcomes. Further research on the intervention dose needed to realize benefit is warranted in this area.

9.4.3 Critical Examination of the Concept of Self-Determination

Several interview participants expressed the opinion that self-determination drives peer support activities, and in their view, assistance in self-management and linkage to clinical care and community resources should generally only be undertaken as they align with the individual's goals. The Mental Health Commission of Canada names self-determination as a core value of peer support [6]. Similarly, the National Association of Peer Supporters in the USA states that peer support is person driven [5]. Both documents hold considerable standing in the field, and certainly, an emphasis on expanding choices rather than constraining them and respecting an individual's choice is a valued aspect of peer support, especially given the historical and ongoing context of coercion in mental health services.

This finding deserves critical and nuanced examination. Firstly, the emphasis placed on self-determination in peer support presents challenges for research. As different people likely will have different goals, defining success or effectiveness of peer support is difficult. Involving peers in the design and conduct of research may lead to innovative approaches to meet this challenge. Furthermore, in contrast to the emphasis on self-determination per se, international peer support experts note that cultural variation calls into question the absolute centrality of the notion of self-determination in peer support, as, for example, people in collectivist cultures tend to cede decision-making power to the elders in their family [31]. In response to such cultural considerations, these experts came together and developed a set of guiding values, principles, and practices as a framework to maintain role integrity while allowing for local adaptation [31]. In the resulting core practices language, these authors assert that peers "support people in taking ownership of their own lives and decisions, even if these decisions involve affording other people important roles in making decisions about their lives" and "focus on those health and quality of life outcomes most important to the people they support" [31].

The concept of self-determination in peer support may also be examined from the perspective of the distinction between nondirective and directive support. The emphasis on autonomy and choice in writing on peer support [32] overlaps considerably with nondirective supports' focus on respecting recipients' choices and preferences. Research on nondirective and directive support, however, reports certain instances in which directive support may be especially helpful, such as in especially challenging circumstances or when someone is overwhelmed with choices [33–36]. For example, reported directive instrumental support, or stepping in and "doing for" someone, was found to be effective in reducing depressive symptoms among people who were socially isolated, while it was not effective among people who were not socially isolated [36]. In the same analyses, however, nondirective emotional support was also associated with fewer depressive symptoms among those who were isolated. That both directive instrumental and nondirective emotional support may be associated with fewer depressive symptoms suggests that these types of support are complementary to each other and not a unidimensional opposition of directive and nondirective, linearly related to mood.

Parallel to seeing nondirective and directive as complementary, a more nuanced approach to the value of self-determination might consider complexities. For example, situations may arise in which recipients of peer support face substantial challenges that overwhelm their resources and for which direct advice and assistance may sometimes be helpful. Certainly, peer support is voluntary, and any action taken is ultimately up to the individual. However, people who are in stressful and overwhelming situations, as many recipients of mental health peer support are, may not be able to identify what might be beneficial without some guidance. At times, a more directive approach may help people better address concrete challenges they face. Through experience, peers may learn in which instances more direction may be helpful and use this knowledge to best support their clients.

9.4.4 Variety and Multiple Models

Finally, and perhaps most importantly, this project did not find evidence for a singular best practice design or approach to peer support. Rather, the realist review identified a plurality of peer programs, and no one approach had a monopoly on documented benefits. As such, results suggest there is room for multiple models of peer support, such as programs that employ peer specialists to deliver support in clinical spaces, illness-specific mutual support groups, and clubhouse models where clients and staff work alongside each other. Careful consideration of the peer support activities, implementation facilitators and barriers, and key challenges suggested here may allow for improved design of many different models. Key steps in program development might be situating the proposed program on the continuum of peer support, from formal to informal; considering the core components of peer support put forth here and providing as many as feasible; and then making adaptations based on the unique considerations of the program's audience and its stated objectives. People who experience psychosis encounter numerous difficulties as they navigate illness, recovery, and life. It follows that they might find benefit in a variety of styles of peer support programs.

References

1. Moll S, Holmes J, Geronimo J, Sherman D. Work transitions for peer support providers in traditional mental health programs: unique challenges and opportunities. Work. 2009;33(4):449–58.
2. Lloyd-Evans B, Mayo-Wilson E, Harrison B, Istead H, Brown E, Pilling S, et al. A systematic review and meta-analysis of randomised controlled trials of peer support for people with severe mental illness. BMC Psychiatry. 2014;14(1):39.
3. Chinman M, George P, Dougherty RH, Daniels AS, Ghose SS, Swift A, et al. Peer support services for individuals with serious mental illnesses: assessing the evidence. Psychiatr Serv. 2014;65(4):429–41. https://doi.org/10.1176/appi.ps.201300244.
4. Asad S. The role of peer support providers in inter-professional mental health care teams. Ottawa: Health Systems: Tefler School of Management, University of Ottawa; 2015.
5. Foglesong D, Knowles K, Cronise R, Wolf J, Edwards JP. National Practice Guidelines for peer support specialists and supervisors. Psychiatr Serv. 2022;73(2):215–8.
6. Cyr C, Mckee H, O'Hagan M, Priest R. Making the case for peer support. Ottawa: Mental Health Commission of Canada; 2016. 2007–16
7. Mead S, Hilton D, Curtis L. Peer support: a theoretical perspective. Psychiatr Rehabil J. 2001;25(2):134.
8. Mead S, MacNeil C. Peer support: what makes it unique. Int J Psychosoc Rehabil. 2006;10(2):29–37.
9. Fisher EB, Ballesteros J, Bhushan N, Coufal MM, Kowitt SD, McDonough AM, et al. Key features of peer support in chronic disease prevention and management. Health Aff. 2015;34(9):1523–30.
10. Evans M, Daaleman TP, Fisher EB. Peer support for chronic medical conditions. In: Avery J, editor. Peer support in medicine: a quick guide. New York: Springer; 2021. p. 49–70.
11. Fisher EB, Boothroyd RI, Coufal MM, Baumann LC, Mbanya JC, Rotheram-Borus MJ, et al. Peer support for self-management of diabetes improved outcomes in international settings. Health Aff. 2012;31(1):130–9.
12. Fisher EB, Earp JA, Maman S, Zolotor A. Cross-cultural and international adaptation of peer support for diabetes management. Fam Pract. 2009;27(suppl_1):i6–i16.
13. Plett H. The art of holding space: a practice of love, liberation, and leadership. Vancouver: Page Two Books, Incorporated; 2020.
14. Aschbrenner KA, Naslund JA, Shevenell M, Kinney E, Bartels SJ. A pilot study of a peer-group lifestyle intervention enhanced with mHealth technology and social media for adults

with serious mental illness. J Nerv Ment Dis. 2016;204(6):483–6. https://doi.org/10.1097/NMD.0000000000000530.
15. Young AS, Cohen AN, Goldberg R, Hellemann G, Kreyenbuhl J, Niv N, et al. Improving weight in people with serious mental illness: the effectiveness of computerized services with peer coaches. J Gen Intern Med. 2017;32(Suppl 1):48–55. https://doi.org/10.1007/s11606-016-3963-0.
16. Kelly EL, Braslow JT, Brekke JS. Using electronic health records to enhance a peer health navigator intervention: a randomized pilot test for individuals with serious mental illness and housing instability. Community Ment Health J. 2018;54(8):1172–9. https://doi.org/10.1007/s10597-018-0282-4.
17. Kelly E, Duan L, Cohen H, Kiger H, Pancake L, Brekke J. Integrating behavioral healthcare for individuals with serious mental illness: a randomized controlled trial of a peer health navigator intervention. Schizophr Res. 2017;182:135–41. https://doi.org/10.1016/j.schres.2016.10.031.
18. V.A. Office of Research and Development. Peer support for exercise in older veterans with psychotic disorders. https://ClinicalTrials.gov/show/NCT02958007 (2021). Accessed 27 May 2020.
19. Penney D. Defining "peer support": implications for policy, practice, and research. 2018.
20. Mirbahaeddin E, Chreim S. A narrative review of factors influencing peer support role implementation in mental health systems: implications for research, policy and practice. Adm Policy Ment Health Ment Health Serv Res. 2022;49:1–17.
21. Mutschler C, Bellamy C, Davidson L, Lichtenstein S, Kidd S. Implementation of peer support in mental health services: a systematic review of the literature. Psychol Serv. 2022;19(2):360.
22. Ibrahim N, Thompson D, Nixdorf R, Kalha J, Mpango R, Moran G, et al. A systematic review of influences on implementation of peer support work for adults with mental health problems. Soc Psychiatry Psychiatr Epidemiol. 2020;55(3):285–93.
23. Glasgow RE, Funnell MM, Bonomi AE, Davis C, Beckham V, Wagner EH. Self-management aspects of the improving chronic illness care breakthrough series: implementation with diabetes and heart failure teams. Ann Behav Med. 2002;24(2):80–7.
24. Pawson R, Greenhalgh T, Harvey G, Walshe K. Realist review-a new method of systematic review designed for complex policy interventions. J Health Serv Res Policy. 2005;10(1_suppl):21–34.
25. Ragin CC. Using qualitative comparative analysis to study causal complexity. Health Serv Res. 1999;34(5 Pt 2):1225.
26. Powers MA, Bardsley J, Cypress M, Duker P, Funnell MM, Hess Fischl A, et al. Diabetes self-management education and support in type 2 diabetes: a joint position statement of the American Diabetes Association, the American Association of Diabetes Educators, and the Academy of Nutrition and Dietetics. Diabetes Care. 2015;38(7):1372–82.
27. Kidd SA, Mutschler C, Lichtenstein S, Yan S, Virdee G, Blair F, et al. Randomized trial of a brief peer support intervention for individuals with schizophrenia transitioning from hospital to community. Schizophr Res. 2021;231:214–20.
28. Chinman MJ, Weingarten R, Stayner D, Davidson L. Chronicity reconsidered: improving person-environment fit through a consumer-run service. Community Ment Health J. 2001;37(3):215–29. https://doi.org/10.1023/A:1017577029956.
29. Weingarten R, Chinman M, Tworkowski S, Stayner D, Davidson L. The welcome basket project: consumers reaching out to consumers. Psychiatr Rehabil J. 2000;24(1):65.
30. Gillard S, Bremner S, Patel A, Goldsmith L, Marks J, Foster R, et al. Peer support for discharge from inpatient mental health care versus care as usual in England (ENRICH): a parallel, two-group, individually randomised controlled trial. Lancet Psychiatry. 2022;9(2):125–36.
31. Stratford AC, Halpin M, Phillips K, Skerritt F, Beales A, Cheng V, et al. The growth of peer support: an international charter. J Ment Health. 2017:1–6. https://doi.org/10.1080/09638237.2017.1340593.
32. Repper J, Aldridge B, Gilfoyle S, Gillard S, Perkins R, Rennison J. Peer support workers: theory and practice. University Park: Citeseer; 2013.

33. Kowitt S, Yu S, Owens AK, Carey LA, Fisher EB. Social support needs among patients with advanced breast cancer: sensitivity trumps substance. J Commun Supportive Oncol. 2016;14(12):509–14.
34. Fisher E, Bickle C, Harber K, Hughes C, Jeffe D, Kahl L, et al. Benefits of directive and non-directive support are moderated by severity of circumstances. Annual meeting of Society of Behavioral Medicine, San Francisco, CA 1997.
35. Gabriele JM, Carpenter BD, Tate DF, Fisher EB. Directive and nondirective e-coach support for weight loss in overweight adults. Ann Behav Med. 2010;41(2):252–63.
36. Evans M, Fisher EB. Social isolation and mental health: the role of nondirective and directive social support. Community Ment Health J. 2021; https://doi.org/10.1007/s10597-021-00787-9.

Index

M. Evans, *Peer Support Services Reaching People with Schizophrenia*, https://doi.org/10.1007/978-3-031-29042-8

MIX
Papier aus verantwortungsvollen Quellen
Paper from responsible sources
FSC® C105338

If you have any concerns about our products,
you can contact us on
ProductSafety@springernature.com

In case Publisher is established outside the EU,
the EU authorized representative is:
Springer Nature Customer Service Center GmbH
Europaplatz 3, 69115 Heidelberg, Germany

Printed by Libri Plureos GmbH
in Hamburg, Germany